After years of working in professions which impose remorseless wear and tear on the skin and hair, international model Pat Wellington and actress Suzy Kendall decided to produce their own fragrant herbal preparations. Their lotions and creams are made of things like strawberries and cucumbers, comfrey and coconut oil, juniper and birch—as well as more exotic things like aloe and jojoba oil.

As well as briefly relating the story of their lives, including their search for new and original herbal cosmetics, Pat and Suzy tell how their small enterprise blossomed into a successful business venture, to the point where their products are now available to the public. They give simple, practical advice on how to make up your own beauty recipes with ingredients found in your window box, garden or even at your local greengrocer, and provide a list of the main herbs they use and recommend.

With the charming line drawings, and the photographs of Pat and Suzy at work and at home, this is a delightfully personal account of the secrets of natural beauty.

Suzy Kendall & Pat Wellington

NATURAL APPEAL

J. M. Dent & Sons Ltd
London, Toronto & Melbourne

We should like to make special thanks to Anthea Disney and Peter Jarvis, B.Sc., for all their help and advice.

First published 1980
© Suzy Kendall and Pat Wellington 1980

Made in Great Britain by
Butler & Tanner Ltd, Frome and London, for
J. M. Dent & Sons Ltd
Aldine House, Welbeck Street, London

British Library Cataloguing in Publication Data

Kendall, Suzy
  Natural appeal.
  1. Beauty, Personal
  2. Diet
  3. Food, Natural
  I. Title   II. Wellington, Pat
  646.7′2   RA778

ISBN 0-460-04525-3

Contents

1 Introduction

When we first met the occasion was not particularly auspicious. We had both been hired as models for a commercial and flown to Jamaica along with six other girls to look glamorous and seductive in the tropical sunshine. We found ourselves sharing a hotel suite, two total strangers accustomed to the transitory friendships forged in the world of modelling.

But what we found on each other's dressing tables was to turn us into allies and, eventually, business partners. For among the paraphernalia that every model hauls around the globe—hot rollers, wigs, makeup and the rest of the tricks of the trade—Pat discovered that Suzy had a large pot of unidentifiable cream that she kept under close guard, and Pat, to Suzy's amazement, was carting around a teapot and a dozen little packets of assorted, fragrant-smelling herbs.

After comparing notes, we soon discovered we shared a reluctance to rely on commercial beauty products. We had both acquired a profound mistrust of them after intensive use in our professions. The rest of our spare time in the West Indies was spent explaining our homegrown beauty remedies to each other.

As the story moved on, Pat's career accelerated her into one of the most successful and enduring models in this country and Suzy went on to become an actress and star of films like *Penthouse*, *Thirty Is A Dangerous Age*, *Cynthia* and *To Sir With Love*.

We continued to stay in touch, swap home remedies and develop our interest in natural beauty products, using just what we had in our kitchens and any herbs we could find which would grow in our gardens. Eventually Suzy was to spend a lot of time in California, where she introduced Pat to more exotic plants like the aloe and the papaya.

In the world of modelling and acting, where harsh light and extreme weather take their toll on women whose looks are all-important, friends began to ask us if they could try our herbal hair rinses and simple skin masks and creams. Soon both our refrigerators were stacked with bottles and jars of sweet-smelling potions that we were making up in growing quantities.

The idea of actually selling our homemade remedies occurred to us again and again, but we were both busy working in our respective areas and neither of us wanted to give up the time needed to perfect and market our ideas: it would need the help of an analytical chemist and would involve finding a factory, packaging, designing, selling and bookkeeping. So the idea remained just that.

Then in 1978 Suzy, who was by now married to commodity trader Sandy Harper, became pregnant. It seemed like the perfect time to make our dream a reality so Pat agreed to arrange her modelling career so that it would allow the two of us to set about planning and organising our now successful natural beauty business, Kendall-Wellington & Co. Ltd.

As it turned out, Suzy's pregnancy was fraught with complications and most of our venture was planned from her hospital bed, where she had to stay for over four months. The sight of Pat, stunningly made up and dressed, arriving straight from a modelling job laden down with samples of bottles and labels, became a common sight to the bewildered nurses and doctors. Suzy, in a hospital room surrounded by filing cabinets and the telephone unable to move, organised everything.

As soon as Suzy's daughter, Elodie, was born, Kendall-Wellington went into business properly, in 1979, and now a refined version of our original beauty remedies is available not just to our friends, but to everyone.

2 Suzy

My first encounter with natural remedies was not what you might call fortuitous. My grandmother, a firm, determined Derbyshire woman from Belper, heard me sneeze a couple of times and put me straight into a hot mustard bath. Not that a teaspoonful is bad for a cold, but my granny was not a woman to do things by halves and she shook in almost the whole tin of mustard which made the water so hot I could barely stand it—or, rather, sit in it—and admonished me to stay there until she gave permission to get out.

Twenty minutes later I was bright red all over and my skin was burning. From then on whenever I had a cold coming on I fled from my grandmother's hearing, into her garden where she grew what to me first looked like a lot of weeds but what was in fact a classic English herb garden. At weekends I'd be pressed unwillingly into service, making pomanders by the dozen and lavender bags by the gross for her huge cupboards and chests of drawers.

Had I known that one day I would be starting a herbal beauty business, I might have taken a little more notice of what my grandmother could have taught me. She would, indeed, have been horrified at my ignorance when I first started making myself a cleansing cream and freshener, struggling to remember what she had done with ease and familiarity all those years before.

As a girl growing up in a Derbyshire village, cosmetics and the sophistication of the fashion industry were about as alien to me as flying to the moon. My beauty routine consisted of washing my face with soap and water and buying whatever shampoo had a pretty label. I managed to emerge from art college and several jobs as a fabric designer with a love for aesthetics, several pairs of jeans and one lipstick.

On one of my rare forays to London an incident was to

occur which would turn my life upside down. I decided to
have my hair done and naturally went to the only hairdresser
that I had seen written about in our local paper, French of
London, where Roy, the unfortunate man delegated to deal
with me, suggested I might have my blonde hair streaked.
On hearing the price I declined with alacrity. Anyway I
thought it would grow out, and I wasn't paying all that
money for something that wouldn't last a good five years.

In the next chair was, quite by chance, Cherry
Marshall, one of the top London model agents, and she told
Roy that if the odd girl who was giving him such a hard time
wanted to do any modelling, she would be happy to take me
on her books. So Roy, bless him, firmly manoeuvred me to
her office next door after my hair was dry, but when Cherry
Marshall explained what she could offer—trips abroad,
commercials, magazine pictures—I was very sceptical. That
whole world was foreign to me and I knew no one who had
ever been involved in it. When Cherry told me I would need
a set of photographs taken of myself so that she could 'sell'
me, I immediately decided that was the catch. She just
wanted to con me into paying for these pictures and that
would be the end of it. I was not a very trusting soul.

Happily Cherry, confronted by this blunt, uninformed
and obstinate young woman, did not do the sensible thing
and dismiss me. She said instead that, as proof of her
goodwill, *she* would pay for the contact sheets—an unheard-
of thing in a world where everyone takes care of themselves
first.

In fact, two days after that first interview she got me a
job doing a TV commercial for toothpaste. Since I'd never
owned a mascara brush let alone a foundation, I was whisked
off to Max Factor where they made me up in the style of the
day, pancake applied all over the face, heavy eyeshadow, eye
liner, false eyelashes, different rouges and tons of powder.

My first shock in the studio was that I was told not to
put the toothpaste on the brush because a mouthful of white
foam is not exactly enticing, so I scrubbed away for hours
with a clean brush. Being short-sighted, I couldn't see the

camera so I wasn't nervous and since all the client demanded was a pretty girl who smiled and had even teeth, it was an auspicious beginning. It was my smile and my teeth that eventually led to my doing 35 commercials. Luckily I seemed to be just right for the girl-next-door look.

My next big job was to spend a month with five other model girls doing a catalogue for the next season's clothes. When I arrived for work I had only the clothes I stood up in and my trusty lipstick. I kept peering short-sightedly and with disbelief at the other girls who had brought hair pieces, boxes of different kinds of cosmetics, hair dryers, heated rollers and special brushes and lacquers. It was obvious to them that I was a novice but, instead of dismissing me, they sat me down and taught me how to make up, shade my face, cover my flaws and generally make the best of myself.

On discovering that I was living at the not exactly trendy Imperial Hotel, because that's where my grandmother had always stayed, several of the models who shared a flat took pity on me and invited me to live with them. It was from them that I learned everything about the business. It was a crash course in my new life.

My only problem in this new and wonderful existence of travel and filming was my skin. Having been accustomed to fresh air and to being washed twice a day, my face was suddenly being covered in heavy cosmetics, subjected to harsh, hot lights, and all it got in the way of care from me was a theatrical cleansing cream. The inevitable occurred, my face started to itch, I would get rashes and eventually my skin became so sensitive that I went to a dermatologist. He told me that my skin merely needed kindness and his advice was not to wear heavy makeup, or if I did, to ensure that it contained no perfumes which would only add to the irritation, and to buy natural products without synthetics added.

The proliferation of health food shops and herbal treatments was yet to come, so finding natural creams and fresheners was almost impossible. I therefore began trying to concoct them in the kitchen at the flat – much to the amazement of the other girls. One valuable piece of advice the doctor had given me was to cleanse my face finally with a solution made of witch hazel, rosewater and distilled water, so I would always carry around my own little creams and lotions to jobs.

I began to travel to places which had merely been names on a map before and the more television commercials I made, the more I became fascinated by acting rather than just posing. So I started a course of acting classes, although it all seemed such a cliché (model turns actress) that I only told my agent.

My new life seemed very exotic. I was spending a great deal of it in beautiful, sunny climates because most commercials demand reliable weather and, of course, the unexpected often happened.

On a hairspray commercial which we filmed in Jamaica, hundreds of extras were brought in to stand around and hide the palm trees in the distance because the scene was meant to take place somewhere in England. We waited for sunset, for the blazing red sky of the Caribbean that comes at that hour, I was dressed in a beautiful long, white dress, the sand of the beach was startingly white and my supposed lover, a male model dressed in a white suit, was to drive me in a long, white Cadillac into the surf as my hair blew enticingly in the breeze.

It all went according to plan, the sky was red, the male model smiled, the cameras turned, my hair blew glamorously into the wind... only unfortunately he was a terrible driver and in his enthusiasm he drove us both too far into the sea. We had to struggle damply back to the beach, our clothes clinging to us, because the car could not be budged.

The next day we went back to the beach to see a bunch of workmen with a crane trying to rescue the car, which by now had sunk so deeply into the sand that only the tip of the white bonnet was visible. It was a hopeless task, we lost a beautiful new Cadillac and some enterprising Jamaicans undoubtedly managed to retrieve a brand-new, if slightly salt-damaged car after we'd gone.

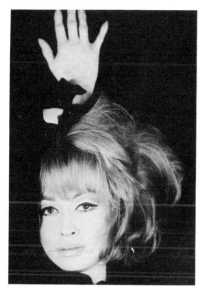

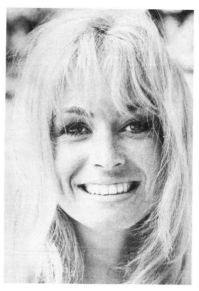

One of my first modelling pictures with heavy makeup (taken by photographer John Cole).

I'm learning to use less makeup, even letting my freckles show for an 'outdoor' look.

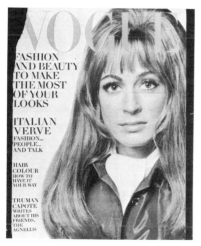

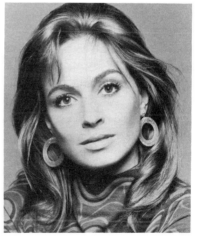

Cover taken by David Bailey for *Vogue*.

For this shot I have had my hair streaked with darker shades to tone down the bleaching from the sun, and am using makeup more subtly (picture by Barry Latigan).

After that job, I decided to take advantage of my free ticket and go to see Montego Bay on the beautiful north shore of Jamaica. Arriving at the deserted airport at midnight, wondering how to find a taxi, I suddenly heard a voice yell 'Suzy'. It was a model girl who had opened a dress shop on the island. I meant to stay a week. I was there three months.

My luck held. As I walked into my London flat after those months of unexplained absence, the phone was ringing. It was my agent, she had an audition for me the next day for a feature film *Up Jumped A Swagman*, in which I was to play Frank Ifield's dream girl. The acting was minimal, all I had to do was look good and pose a lot. After three readings and two screen tests I got the job and I was, finally, an actress— of sorts.

I learned fast. Immediately after that film, I got a part in *The Liquidator*, a picture Rod Taylor and Trevor Howard were making in the same studios at Pinewood. I was also learning that the beauty problems an actress faces rarely occur so drastically in real life. No one else would spend two weeks in a 'tank' of chlorinated water for underwater photography, or be expected to cry for hours until their eyes are red and sore, if not from the tears themselves, from the ammonia wafted under their noses to continue the flow. No one else is subjected to such a barrage of lights, or constant re-touching of makeup, particularly of powder—so that no moisture or sweat, which is ever-present, caused by the heat of the lights, will show in the finished film. I think makeup women and men must get through tons of the stuff. I know my face at the end of the day was often caked solid. All this because even a few minutes finished film can take weeks to produce.

Anyway, the excitement of completing that second film made me decide to celebrate, so I went off to the sun and lazed luxuriously on a beach for two weeks until I had a call from the studio—they wanted me back immediately for an extra close-up. I duly arrived at Pinewood only to see horror on the face of the makeup man. I had made the film with my normal, pale complexion but now my skin was a dark shade of coffee.

I was sent to lie down for two hours with a mask of yoghurt on my face (a tip I have since used when my greed for the sun has made me foolhardy), so that the brightness from my exposure to the sun would calm down. Chastened, I returned to have the makeup artist paint my face and neck with pale theatrical foundation, again and again, until he had disguised my suntan enough to do the shot. I had learned my first lesson: actors—and especially actresses—cannot afford to get a tan unless they are well and truly between films.

Despite the tips I had picked up (by now I could actually manage to do a proper makeup job on myself), when I wasn't working I still dressed in jeans and went without cosmetics. My theatrical agent, Dennis Selinger, got me an audition for the TV series *Mogul*, and asked me to change my image and look sexy, which was what the part called for.

So I carefully dressed myself, put my straight and difficult hair on rollers, covered it with a scarf and planned to comb it out and put the finishing touches to my makeup in the ladies' cloakroom just before I had to face the producers. Everything went according to plan, I had managed to cover up my Derbyshire accent by taking voice classes, I was dressed to kill, and I'd remembered to take off my glasses, as Dennis had told me to do.

The door to the audition room opened and I could just see the forms of seven men sitting round a table, so with my best smile forward I walked up to them with what I hoped was a mixture of sexuality and confidence. What I couldn't see without my glasses was that one man had his foot sticking out, so they were all treated to the sight of this new property falling flat on her face, saying 'oh bloody 'ell' in an accent that was anything but classless. My handbag which contained all my hair rollers not to mention a host of other unglamorous items tipped all over the floor and before anyone could stop laughing I'd picked myself up and retreated with a burning face into a taxi and home. Needless to say, I didn't get that part, but my luck still held.

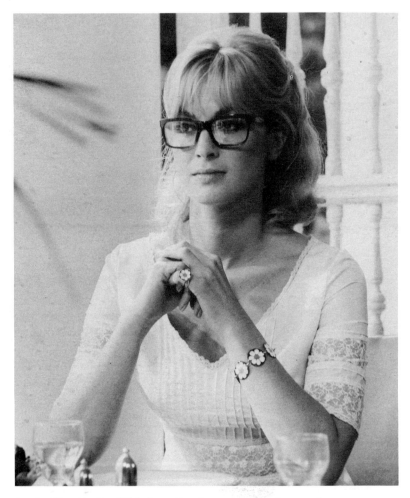

In the film *To Sir With Love*, I at last wore my glasses—but to my dismay they took out my lenses and put in clear glass. Optical glass distorts the eyes on film—so I was still short-sighted. (Columbia Pictures)

The writer of the series, who'd been sitting at the table and witnessed the whole thing, wrote an episode specially for me entitled *Meet Miss Mogul* about a girl from the Midlands who is made to take off her glasses and manages to fall clumsily over everything, including her own feet.

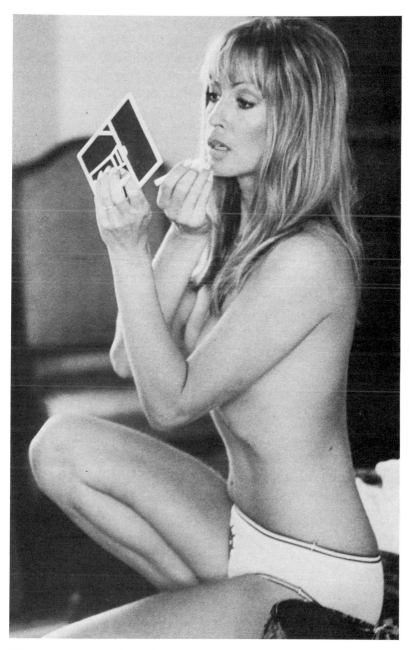

The ever-present makeup mirror (taken by Chiara Samugheo in Rome).

Despite being accident-prone, my career was flourishing. I made *To Sir With Love* with Sidney Poitier, *Thirty Is A Dangerous Age*, *Cynthia* with my then-husband Dudley Moore, *Penthouse* with Terence Morgan, *Up The Junction* with Dennis Waterman, *Fear is the Key* with Barry Newman and a host of other pictures all over the world, from Los Angeles to Dubrovnik.

My only real problem seemed to be coping with my complexion and hair, both of which needed coddling to survive not only the rigours of filming, but also the off set publicity shots. Believe me, most of these pictures captioned 'between film takes' are decidedly not as you really look. I seemed to be most of the time in rollers so that my hair would look the same from take to take and day to day. Often my stunt man in my blonde wig looked better than I did.

In a film called *Fraulein Doktor* I played a woman spy with eight different disguises, which meant eight different makeups, wigs and hairstyles. For one character, the makeup man had to give me oriental eyes. Before he put on the wig, he made tiny, painfully tight pin curls all round my hair line. Over my head he then put the top of a nylon stocking attaching it by even more pins to the hair line. Then he pulled the stocking hard and tight, fixing it to the crown. It certainly lifted my eyes and most of my face, too, and by the end of the film some of my hair had been pulled out by the roots and the rest of it broke from the strain.

For six months I couldn't use hot rollers or even a hair dryer, all I could do was eat brewers' yeast tablets, which really do help to strengthen the new hair, and twice weekly use a hot oil treatment (see our recipes) shown me by a makeup lady, who also taught me a trick for puffy eyes caused by excessive 'film' crying. Soak two pads of cotton wool in the juice of a quarter of a cucumber mixed with two teaspoonfuls of witch hazel and place on closed eyes for fifteen minutes—it's fantastic.

I don't want to give the impression that all you need to be an actress is a pretty face and good skin—though they can help. Acting is a skilled craft and for me this makes it a joy.

Pictures from *Fraulein Doktor*—four of eight 'disguises' which I had to adopt as the spy of the title. (Paramount Pictures)

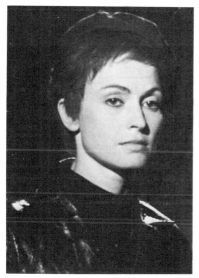

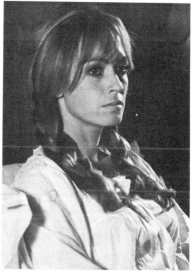

Playing a boy, with no makeup at all and a very, very short wig.

With my own blonde hair plaited for the part of a French maid.

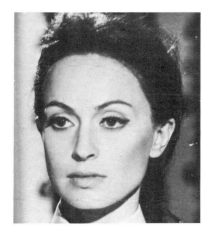

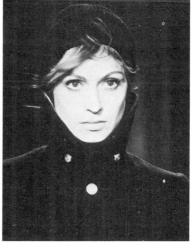

As a Spanish countess. My eyes are pulled up with a stocking under the black wig, which is then stuck down to my hair line.

With a short blonde wig as Fraulein Doktor herself.

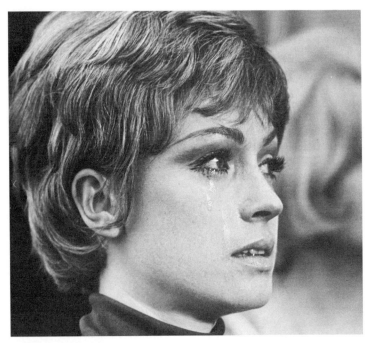

Wearing a short red wig for *Up the Junction*. (Paramount Pictures)

I love losing myself in unreal situations and I can release
emotions which if I indulged in them in real life, would
result in me being locked away. The camaraderie on a film
set is unique—all those people cut off from the rest of the
world, often for months at a time. Oddly, the more horrific
and morbid the story of the film, the jollier the atmosphere
and the more that people seem to need to play practical jokes
on each other.

When I was making *Assault*, a horror film, there was a
scene in which I was meant to be driving a car with a back
projection behind me to give the illusion of moving. Between
every take the makeup man would come over to where I was
sitting alone in the middle of the studio in my 'car' and take
away the shine around my nose and mouth and reapply any
extra powder or lip gloss that was needed. Everyone seemed
to be laughing at one point and I couldn't understand why—

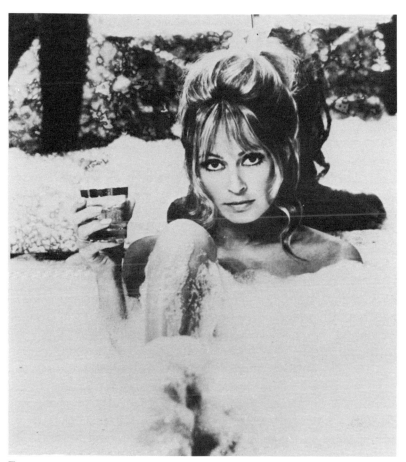

From the film *Darker than Amber*—drinking 'champagne' that was
really cold tea, and immersed in bubbles. (Courtesy of Cinema Center
Films)

my acting maybe! It wasn't until I saw the 'rushes' (the
evening showing of what has been shot the day before) that I
realised why. The shots of me driving the car came up and
suddenly there I was in one take, sporting a black moustache.
The makeup man had painted this on with a so-called
application of powder and cunningly wiped it off with
another—and, without a mirror, I was the only one in the
entire studio not to know what was going on literally under
my nose.

Friendships made in situations like this have an intensity that comes from being together for several weeks or even months from the moment at dawn when you arrive in the cavernous, hangar-like building which is a film studio until evening when the day's work is completed and the rushes have been viewed. Yet, like the plot of the film, many of these friendships end suddenly. But for the time you are together, the cast and the crew create a rapport between themselves which is unique.

This commitment is one of the things I like best about filming and I love the elation I experience when a scene goes well. Acting is not normal work and its compensations, like its demands, are extraordinary.

On one film, *The Gamblers*, the company rented a White Russian's villa for me, built in the Czarist era outside Dubrovnik, with two swimming pools and a bathroom so hedonistic that in addition to the sunken bath, hip bath, foot pool and a loo on a massive raised platform, there was even a special tall, thin pedestal basin just for cleaning your teeth. In the movie, I had to have a sun tan so I was actually paid just to lie by one or other of the pools.

On *Darker than Amber*, filmed in Miami, Florida, I was submerged in a bubble bath for two days, which on a movie set means sitting in detergent while a hosepipe placed strategically under you keeps the pressure up and the bubbles bubbling—otherwise after a few hours of hot lights there'd be no bubbles. When the scene was finally complete, I was dried out and wrinkled like a prune and I spent 24 hours in my hotel room covered in almond oil to try to counteract the effect.

The only time I have ever been called upon to do a nude scene was in *Penthouse* but there was no way I could take my clothes off with a crew of around 50 people watching. So I made myself a costume out of stockinette, shaped like a strapless swimsuit with no sides, which I stuck on with three inch wide surgical bandages. The director, Peter Collinson, brought me out onto the set covered in a towel and everyone knew this was the big scene and there was a strange quiet

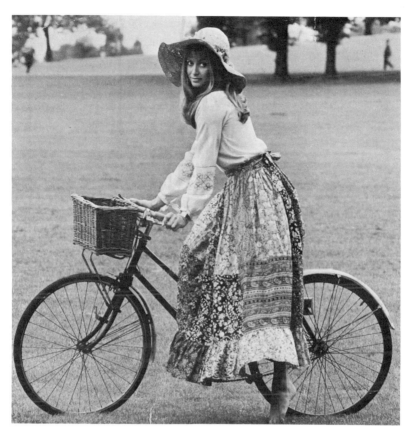

An off-set picture, in which I was meant to look leisurely. In fact I had been working in a short wig only minutes before and it required yet another makeup change for this shot (taken by Brian Aris).

instead of the usual hum of voices. I felt really nervous and Peter sat me down on the bed and said: 'Now Suzy's going to do her rape scene. Unfortunately, I have to tell you she's cut her finger ...' and with that he whipped off my towel, displaying this odd costume I'd made for myself. The effect was wonderful, the uneasiness was immediately diffused and everyone—including me—broke up. What was even better was that my co-star, Tony Beckley, demanded he have a similar outfit and we both ended up taped together because the bandages got stuck!

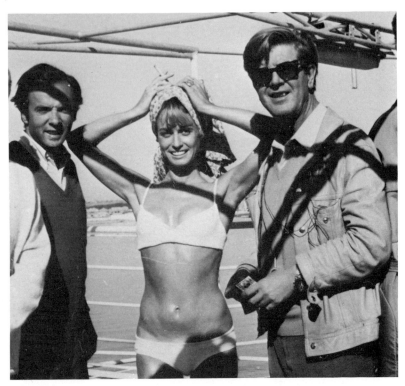

With, left to right, director Ron Winston and Yugoslav lighting cameraman Tomislav. On location aboard ship—I'm trying hard to cover up the fact that I have rollers under my scarf.

After *Penthouse* I played the victim in four other films, a type of character which couldn't be more different from my own. But because I'm smallish, blonde and seemingly fragile that's how I was cast. I must admit it was a relief, and satisfying, when I was asked to appear in a film called *The Bitter End*. The reason? I was finally to get a taste of sweet revenge. I played a murderess.

My career with modelling and films, although hard work, really began through sheer good luck, which seems to have continued to play a great part in my life. Maybe having my daughter Elodie, which was a major factor in making me take time off from filming, will prove as lucky for me in the beauty business that Pat and I have set up.

3 Pat

I was dressed up in a Nell Gwynn outfit, carrying a huge basket which contained not oranges but Walls pork sausages and it was my lot to give them away in Hyde Park for a promotion campaign. Can you imagine what it's like going up to lovers rolling around in the grass and saying, 'Excuse me, but do you want some Walls pork sausages?'

That was my first job from a modelling agency and it was an unforgettable start. I was doing a commercial course at the French Lycée and destined to spend a year in Lille, when I really wanted to study French Literature in Paris. So one day I was sitting at the kitchen table, leafing through the magazine *Vanity Fair* when my eye caught sight of a competition to become named a 'model of the following year'. In those days I had blonde hair that I could sit on and I suddenly thought that, if nothing else, entering the competition would be more exciting than doing my French homework.

I won and the prize was the choice between a modelling course or a 'charm' course at the Lucy Clayton School. Since I still intended to finish my commercial French diploma, I thought 'Well, I don't particularly want to become a model but I might as well have a go at being charming', so I did that 4-week course during my school holidays. But Lucy Clayton's was not particularly thrilled when I announced I was returning to the Lycée and they asked me to show gratitude and do the odd job, which accounts for me trying to give away pork sausages in Hyde Park to people with things on their minds other than breakfast.

Gradually the jobs increased and my interest in the Lycée diminished until I told the principal that I would be leaving. My parents weren't too happy with me, particularly when I told them I'd decided to become a model, but I sold them on the idea that I'd perfect my French if I went to Paris. So I packed my bags, said goodbye to Crystal Palace, the South London suburb where I'd grown up, and set out with fairly good French, a lot of optimism and, of course, a notion of how to be 'charming' which I'd learned at Lucy Clayton's.

I think I learned more in that year I spent in Paris than in all the preceding ones but my charm course was not needed. Within weeks I had a contract with *Elle* magazine to model the collections, the big prize for any new model. I have never forgotten the changing room at *Elle*. It was full of girls but only one of them, an American, would even speak to me. The rest, who were French with a vengeance, did not like foreigners coming in and being snapped up by the magazines, so they totally ostracised me. Once I remember sitting in the dressing room with the American model, playing cards to pass the time while we waited, and one of the French girls came up, deliberately picked up my makeup sponge and began obsessively prodding it with a hairgrip, over and over until the sponge was in shreds. Then, without a word, she dropped the sponge in my lap and walked away.

After a year in Paris I decided to try America and working in New York seemed a breeze. I was taken on by the prestigious Eileen Ford agency and within days was doing a fashion layout at the Hearst mansion in San Simeon, California. I did well in New York in both photographic modelling and television. When I decided to return to London, all that New York and Paris experience paid off. My career took off.

People have strange ideas about models and modelling. They are aware of certain superstars—Twiggy, Lauren Hutton, Jean Shrimpton—but in reality there are a group of girls—20 or 30 usually, at any one time, who are actually doing the bulk of the work i.e. women's magazine work, TV commercials, and catalogue. There used to be terrific snobbery about not doing catalogue work. This now has broken down because of the economic climate, and girls are

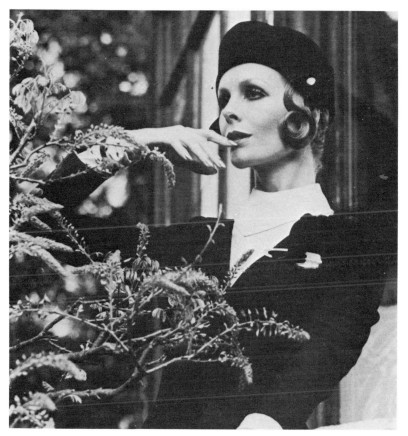

Just one of *nine* changes of clothes and makeup I had to do in two days, for a European makeup campaign. (Photographer, Thomas Cugini. Courtesy Binella Cosmetics, Switzerland)

clamouring to do it. I always have done catalogue work, and am eternally grateful to the 'Littlewoods' and 'Grattans' of this world.

I decided early on that I was interested in modelling as a career which meant one thing—I had to endure in a business not known for its fidelity to anyone. So I assessed myself as objectively as possible. At five feet seven I am a good height for most fashion work and I don't tower over male models, I am blonde which is ideal for advertising because it's seen as being clean and healthy, and perhaps my

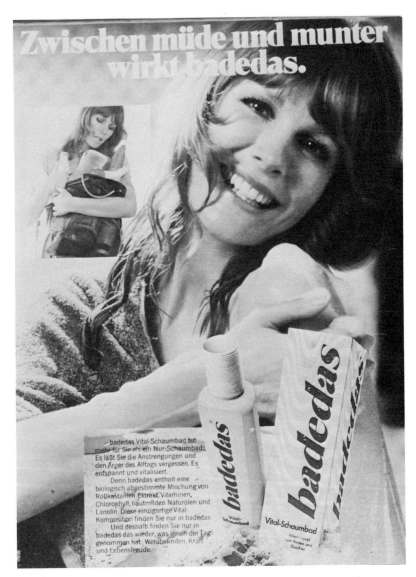

Chiswick for two hours in the morning for this Badedas advertisement, then a rush to the *Sunday Times* studio for a magazine feature that over-ran its time, then to a third appointment at which, at the end of the day, I was supposed to look normal! (Taken by Fred Stundel. Courtesy Beecham Proprietaries)

greatest asset is that I have an adaptable face that can look anything from high fashion to girl-next-door. I was lucky. I fitted into this group of twenty or thirty working girls. But as a model, no matter how successful you may be, you are always aware that instead of building a brilliant career, you are sitting on a diminishing asset. There is no such thing as job security.

There are, of course, times when modelling seems repetitive, boring and plain uncomfortable. But it is a life that has given me terrific freedom and the chance to travel all over the world, from Nepal to Marrakesh and, I have found that, if you can cope with the insecurities and the discomfort of modelling furs in hot weather and bikinis when there's snow on the ground, the rewards are worth the problems. So many people believe that to be a model you have to sell your soul, not to mention a few other things. The truth is that professionalism, reliability and stamina are what persuade people to book you for jobs again and again.

I love to travel but I hate being a tourist so modelling has given me the ideal combination, it has taken me to unlikely places where I have worked for weeks on end and so have really got to know the people and the countries. But, I have to confess, there is another appealing factor in all this: most advertising and magazine work that needs sunshine is shot in the winter, so that it is ready to use when summer arrives in Britain. And spending January or February in the Bahamas is not exactly unpleasant.

I can remember standing in a tent in Marrakesh, swathed in chiffon from head to toe, surrounded by Moroccan bands and dancers and fire-eaters for a Fry's Turkish Delight commercial. I've also seen Rome courtesy of Peter Stuyvesant cigarettes, spent a weekend in Mykonos for Kent cigarettes, cruised the Caribbean for P and O and been one of twelve models chosen from five different countries to be flown to the Canary Islands for just one day—pretty heady and indulgent stuff.

The big test for any model is turning 30, after that anyone unusual-looking seems to bite the dust. I am lucky in

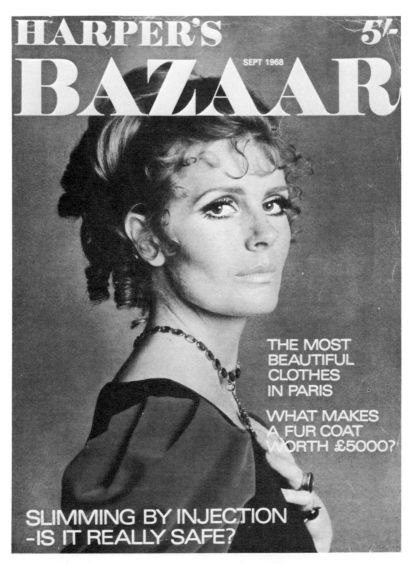

HARPER'S BAZAAR

SEPT 1968

5/-

THE MOST
BEAUTIFUL
CLOTHES
IN PARIS

WHAT MAKES
A FUR COAT
WORTH £5000?

SLIMMING BY INJECTION
-IS IT REALLY SAFE?

Twelve years ago, for *Harper's Bazaar* (*UK*), I think I looked older, with all that makeup on, than I do now. (National Magazine Company Ltd)

that I can look like a young mum yet I can also look classic enough to do those car, drink and travel commercials that are meant to appeal to the sophisticated woman. But after 30, your trendy days are over and you have to accept that you will gradually hear the phone ringing less often as new, younger models are found. Many girls give up at this point but I decided to keep working as much as I could whilst opening my eyes to other avenues of interest.

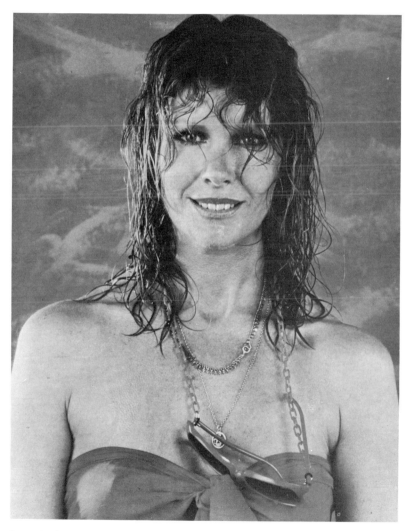

I particularly like this recent shot because, in contrast to the *Harper's* cover, I look healthier and younger than I did then. (Taken by Peter Smith, Scaioni Studios)

Gradually, from my early days in modelling, I had developed a fascination with hair and skin care. At first it was necessity, because, by the nature of my job, I had to know more than other people and I had to cope with beauty problems that are not common to the average English woman.

Gradually, too, I became discontented with most proprietary brands on the market and I was always in search of products that were ultra mild and pure so I began to dabble with herbs, making up a few of my own recipes. My interest really began with a disaster. I was making a commercial for an American hair colourant. At the end of the day's shoot, the chemicals they had used on my hair had, I realised with horror, made it turn a nasty greenish shade and, what's more, it started falling out by the handful. For me it was the end: no hair, no work. So I went to see a hair specialist who had great faith in herbal remedies and he suggested I regularly use birch, burdock and comfrey rinses on my hair to give it back some life and shine and he also gave me some other treatments.

I started visiting friends in Dorset at weekends and I would pick the herbs growing in the hedgerows, steal my friends' cucumbers from the garden and have a field day in the kitchen experimenting with different combinations and trying out old recipes I found in library books.

As a child I had, like Suzy, spent a lot of time with my grandmother and she had always rinsed my hair with rainwater and made infusions of camomile which she said brightened my blonde hair in the summer. I remember once in my early teens I had read some herbal recipe at my grandmother's house for turning hair darker and I'd decided I'd like to be a dramatic brunette. So unknown to my granny I diluted some elderberry juice and poured it over my head which had the unfortunate effect of turning my fair hair a rather blotchy purple. It didn't please my grandmother very much, either.

As I experimented with different herbs I remembered that as a child I had made little muslin bags filled with all

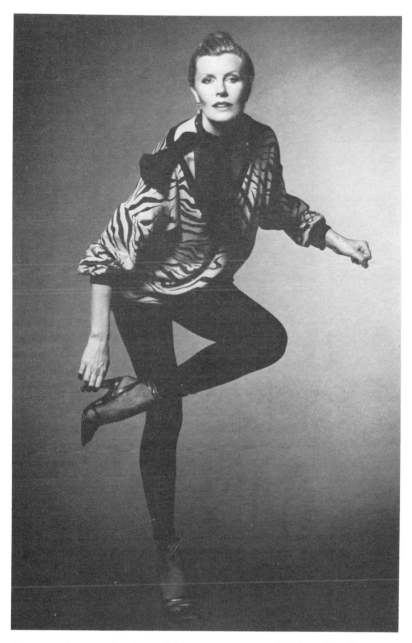

A recent photograph of me which contrasts well with the others here.
(Taken by Mike Martin)

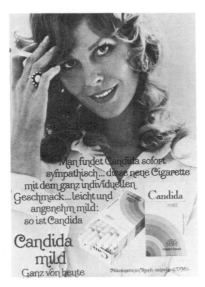

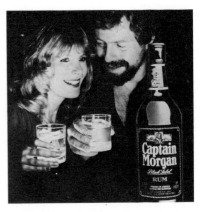

You have to be over 30 to do cigarette advertisements in Germany. This was for a big poster campaign recently—yet another hairstyle! (Courtesy Charlotte Marsh)

We spent two days in August 1979 making this advertisement. On a boiling hot day there was an intense fire burning in the background. The poor dog next to it panted all day long—then it was cut out of the shot, much to our annoyance. (Photographer, Richard Brain. Courtesy Offord Youlten & Associates Ltd)

the good things that grew in profusion in my granny's garden, which we used to hang from the bath taps to scent the water, so I decided to find out all I could about herbs and start making as many products as possible myself.

I once did a show for Helena Rubinstein with a group of other models including Marie Helvin and Joanna Lumley and we were all given very freaky hairstyles and the makeup artist, Christine Skivens, gave me a really eccentric and wonderful coral-coloured face, with crescent moons painted on my cheeks. It was all a lot of fun but, unfortunately for me, I had an appointment for a test for three weeks' work for a rather staid fashion company only half an hour after the Rubinstein show.

There was no way I'd get the job with coral crescents on my face and my hair all frizzed out so, as everyone else stood around after the show drinking champagne, they were

treated to the sight of me emerging from the ladies' room
with wet hair tucked into a towel and my very sophisticated
makeup completely ruined by putting my head under the tap.
Luckily for me, the makeup artist took pity on my
disaster of a face and helped sort me out. She also gave me a
recipe for a good treatment to give my face when I got home
to soften and soothe it after the effects of the day. She told
me to cut holes for the eyes and mouth in a piece of fine
gauze, dip it in warm almond oil, squeeze out the excess and
put the mask flat on my face while I lay down for 20
minutes. Then she told me to massage my face for ten
minutes with little circular movements to remove any dead
skin cells and to finish by removing any unabsorbed oil with
rosewater and witch hazel. This valuable piece of advice has
saved my skin on many occasions and once, after it had
been—literally—sandblasted I spent an entire day applying
the mask, over and over again, to try to get my skin back to
normal.

That was the time I was making a deodorant
commercial in South Africa. I had to stand on top of a huge
sand dune in a white toga, immaculately made up, arms
outstretched, while the director swooped down in a helicopter
to take the shots. But every time he got close enough to get
me in frame, the downdraft from the helicopter whirled what
seemed like the entire sand dune into my face, sticking to my
lipstick, getting on my eyes and smudging my eye makeup.
So we would take one shoot and then I'd trek off to a van
and clean off the sand and reapply the makeup in the mirror.
This went on all day and I had to smile ecstatically even
though, by four in the afternoon, I felt like I didn't have any
skin left on my face and shoulders.

Lack of comfort is one of the hallmarks of modelling.
When I was photographed for a Captain Morgan Rum
Christmas poster it was actually August and boiling hot in
the studio which had a fire burning to make it seem cosy and
warm. By the fire there was a labrador and the poor animal
was panting like crazy but he didn't budge for the entire two
days of shooting. I was really upset when I saw the final

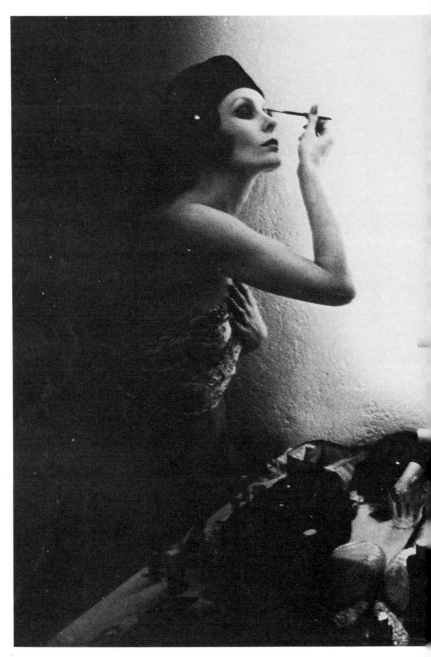

Typical studio dressing room chaos. (Photographer, Thomas Cugini)

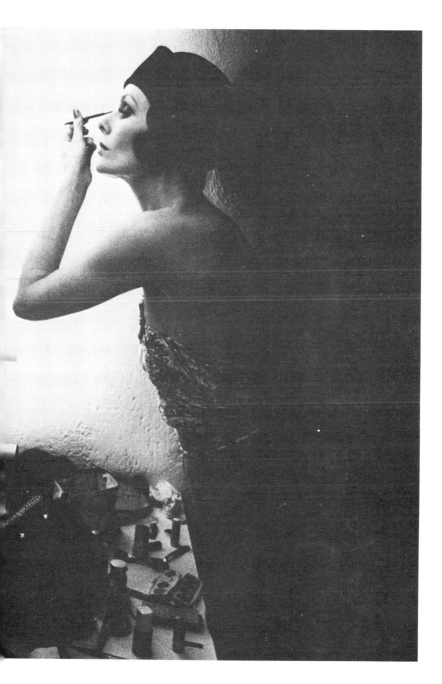

poster and realised the dog had been cut out of the picture—
all that suffering for nothing!

One day I had a two-hour booking in a studio in
Chiswick for a Badedas advert and I had to wear almost no
makeup and have my hair wringing wet. Then I had half an
hour to get to the *Sunday Times* studio where Mike
Berkofsky was shooting a picture of me in which one side of
my face and hair had to be done in the style of Marilyn
Monroe and the other half of my face was to look like
Brigitte Bardot. At 3.30 p.m. I had another booking in
Chelsea where I was to look like a young wife and mother.
At ten to three, after a lot of technical problems, we hadn't
even started shooting my two-sided face so the moment Mike
had finished, I jumped in the car and with my weird face
drove like a maniac to the next appointment. I rushed in the
door only to see the client get one glimpse of my makeup and
nearly pass out with shock.

I was lucky enough to do two Dubonnet commercials.
In the first, which was shot in Italy, I had to drive up to a
beautiful palazzo in an Alfa Romeo dressed in furs, jewellery
and a long white dress. Then I had sexily to drop each item
I was wearing, as I walked up the steps to the palazzo, and as
I got to the top step and began to slide off my dress you
heard this man's voice saying 'make sure the Dubonnet she's
drinking is yours'. In fact, modelling being what it is, the last
shot was done on the steps of the Albert Memorial because it
rained continuously in Italy!

I was very nervous about my second Dubonnet
commercial which was a year later. For the first time I had to
speak several lines of dialogue and I had heard that Ridley
Scott, the director who recently made the film *Alien*, didn't
have much time for people who messed up their scenes. And
I was also working with an actor, supposedly my lover, who
was very patronising about my inexperience.

So there I was all done up in a beautiful dress and in
an elegant setting and I managed to get through it all right.
But at the end of the day, the patronising actor, who had
been sitting drinking Dubonnet all day and waiting for his

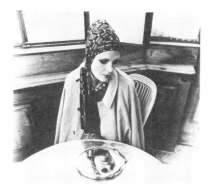

The 'reality' behind the glossy façade—sitting around in a chiffon sleeveless dress on a freezing April day, with somebody's old 'mac' thrown over my shoulders, and bored, waiting for the light to become right!
(Photographer, Thomas Cugini)

turn, was pie-eyed and couldn't get his two lines out!

For this commercial my hair had to be very full and Simon Thompson, the hairdresser, taught me a trick that is the best I've ever come across. He set my hair on very tiny wire rollers then, when it was dry and the rollers were out, he put my head between my knees and brushed the hair from the base of the neck to the ends. Next he told me to throw my head back and shake it gently from side to side so the hair fell into a natural shape but remained very full.

The same hairdresser also told me that he never uses any hair dressings or pommades to smooth out any frizzy or split ends; instead, he rubs a little moisturiser into his hands and then onto the hair. It works better because it's not as greasy as the usual hair cream.

Dubonnet commercials are probably how most people imagine models live all the time. If only they knew. Actually, working with the best directors in beautiful settings with elegant clothes is something we all cherish when it does happen. More often than not you find yourself sitting on a bus for three weeks in non-stop drizzle in Yorkshire, modelling summer dresses when spring has not even arrived. When that last happened to me I decided all nine of us models had two choices—we could sit and look at the rain or we could try and improve ourselves. So we decided on the latter course and I got them all doing yoga exercises and soaking their fingernails in almond oil while we waited for the rain to stop.

Gradually I've noticed how natural products have become a matter of fascination for a lot of other people. Whereas the models I worked with early on frequently thought I was crazy to fiddle around with herbs, now they want to know how to do it themselves. When I went to Greece and learned about yoghurt masks, quite a few of my friends wanted to try it out when they saw me slapping it on. Last summer I was doing some fashion shots and there were flies all over the place but I managed to keep them away from me by wearing a straw hat which had an elder infusion rubbed around the rim. That tip I'd picked up working in Australia, where they have the worst flies I've ever come across.

A Swiss cosmetic company booked me for a campaign which was to demonstrate the wide range of their products. In two days I was made up nine very different ways, from the deeply tanned Peruvian peasant-look to the dramatic chalky-white look of a woman from the film *The Damned*. The poor makeup artist was so worried about my skin suffering from all the different cosmetics he was using and the intense heat of the studio that he made up a wonderful mask for me which he said should replenish the moisture. He took a ripe peach which he peeled and then put in a blender with three tablespoonfuls of peach kernel oil and made me lie down for 20 minutes while the mixture was on my face and neck. After he'd cleaned it off with warm water, my skin felt really soft and not at all irritated.

Being a model is a very double-edged life. We travel and meet people and work hard and have a public image which is very glamorous, but at the end of the day most models go home to a sense of paranoia, the fear that it is all going to end and they will have to strike out and find another way to make a living. I used to think it was like trying to decide what to do when you left school with no qualifications for the outside world.

But modelling has also taken me into another world— the natural beauty business. Slowly but surely it has evolved to the point where I can wake up in the morning and no longer wonder what lies in store for me when I leave school.

4 Starting the Business

Model and actress friends were always asking us to make up an extra batch of bath oils or masks until our refrigerators began to be filled with row after row of pots and bottles and there was barely room to get any food inside.

We knew we could go no further by cooking things up in our kitchens, so when a friend recommended we see an analytical chemist named Peter Jarvis, we were very enthusiastic about the idea. One of the products we took him was the aloe cream Suzy had been making since a visit to Hawaii, and we asked if he could give us his opinion about having it made up in large enough amounts to sell it to our friends and acquaintances who kept asking us for some more.

Peter Jarvis's first response was 'ugh' when he saw our original recipe. He said he was sure it was very effective but instead of boiling up dried aloe leaves we ought to use standardised aloe extract so that the results would be consistent. We would also need to use a different oil as the one we had been working with smelt too heavy in his view, and a lanolin derivative would have to replace the ordinary lanolin we had been using because in some people that causes allergic reactions.

By this point both of us had reached the conclusion that we wanted to sell our products so when Peter also offered to introduce us to Richard Collard, who owns a small factory that makes up natural products in West Sussex, we agreed with alacrity. Previously we had tried talking to major suppliers who made preparations in huge vats for large cosmetic companies but our requirements—that the products contain almost no synthetics and that everything would have to be produced in small quantities—were impracticable for factories of this size. As we were trying to work out the price of 500 pots of moisturiser, orders for hundreds of thousands of pounds would be telephoned into the factory from Italy and France. We realised we were out of our league and, for a while, we gave up hope of finding a factory suited to our scale.

Richard Collard later told us our arrival on his doorstep was a mixed blessing. He was expecting us to be one of those clients who only have a vague idea of what they want from a product and even leave the packaging and naming of the various creams and lotions to him. Instead, he was suddenly confronted by two determined young women with very firm ideas of how each preparation should smell, look, feel on the skin and appear to the user.

Of course, we often took our ideas to be tested without knowing what the ingredients should be for commercial use and without knowing the language of the beauty business. The technical terms were quite beyond us. But Richard Collard and Peter Jarvis were, we have to say, incredibly patient with us, not even complaining when we sent a body lotion back *nine* times for minute changes in viscosity, colour, scent and so on.

We also had limited capital for the development of our products but we wanted the highest quality with the most visual appeal because we felt our names should be on each jar and pot and we had no intention of hiding behind a company.

Our final decision was to put our money into the products themselves and to keep the packaging and labelling as simple as possible. After all, we had often complained about those elaborate little jars we had bought which had fake bottoms, as a result of which one ended up paying a fortune for a pretty jar and very little cream.

We decided on clear, light plastic bottles for the liquids because we both travel a lot and know how much easier it is with a lightweight container. The only time we would use a glass bottle, we decided, was for a perfume or an after-shave lotion because the perfume evaporates through plastic. We even looked at over 200 different samples until we found one that was easy to hold, a good largish size and looked plain but attractive. Then we had to find good, clean white lids and screw tops, with sprinklers inside when necessary, because both of us had so frequently encountered tops that broke or split or simply were not watertight. During the early stages of our formation, we had to decide on a firm policy regarding the use of preservatives. Since unpreserved preparations will have a short shelf-life due to attack by micro-organisms it was obvious that some means of preservation was essential. However, there exists no such thing as a natural preservative (and we wished to have entirely natural products) and furthermore some preservatives can, if used injudiciously, cause allergic reaction. The reader will appreciate that we were faced with a predicament that had no easy solution.

Eventually we decided to compromise by using preservatives at a concentration only high enough to inhibit the growth of undesirable organisms. This involved frequent and prolonged trials during development to get the quantity just right, but in this way we maintained, as high as possible, the content of natural raw materials.

Since our business was going to be mail order at first we felt we should keep the labels simple and send out a small brochure which would describe all the products. Here we had a small headache, for there are government rules and regulations which apply to what you can call a cream and as to where you list its weight on the packaging. We learned, for example, that we couldn't sell an 'anti-wrinkle' cream but we could call it a 'wrinkle' cream. The stringent laws covering beauty products are, of course, necessary for the consumer's protection, but for two people accustomed to wearing aprons and whipping things up at home, it was an unexpected complication.

As an actress and a model we were lucky when it came to launching ourselves, our names were known and our journalist friends were helpful in getting beauty writers to try our creams, and if they liked them to do a piece about us. Luckily we gained quite a lot of publicity, and we went into business officially in September 1979. We now operate the business from 1, Balfour Place, London W1.

Now we still struggle over the book-keeping, the VAT and the banking, but we make a point of personally answering all the letters we receive asking for help or information. Each package that leaves us bears a personal message and many, you may be surprised to hear, are in reply to men who have written in for our products; perhaps the most successful one from the man's point of view is our moisturiser, which is perfect for an after-shaving balm. Now, however, we are venturing into shops and are even starting a special line of beauty preparations for men and we may, of course, find that they appeal to women as well.

5 In the Kitchen

Basic kitchen equipment is all that is necessary to make up
most homemade recipes. You will need:

2–3 stainless steel saucepans
1 very small pan for warming tiny amounts (although
you can manage with a larger pan)
1 pudding basin to use as a bain-marie, or a double
saucepan. (We have found that a pudding basin placed
inside a larger pan, just as you would cook a Christmas
pudding, works fine.)
1 set of measuring spoons
1 pestle and mortar
1 measuring cup
1 blender, a wooden spoon and a strong wrist. (An
electric blender is not for creams as it puts too much
air into them.)
1 sieve
1 small strainer
1 container with a lid for infusions (it has to be able to
stand boiling water so we both use an old teapot)
1 funnel
1 jug or pot to hold strained infusions
A selection of jars, tubs, pots with lids. You can
actually use just about any container but both of us like
to scout the junk shops and pick up pretty old bottles
and jars for a few pence. It makes no difference to
the contents but it makes *us* feel better. Also, try to
find dark pots and jars, as the contents will last longer
out of the light.
Labels—essential as you will forget afterwards what is
in those little jars.
Earthenware pots with lids for long periods of steeping.

Weights and Measures

These can be confusing since weight is different from volume in terms of measurement. Roughly speaking, the following list will work as equivalents for you in the kitchen:

65 drops = 1 teaspoon
3 teaspoons = 1 tablespoon
2 tablespoons = $\frac{1}{8}$ cup = 1 fl. oz.
16 tablespoons = 1 cup = 8 fl. oz.

65 drops = 5 ml = 1 teaspoon
1000 mls = 1 litre
1 litre = 1.759 pints
1 pint = 20 fl. oz. = 0.568 litres

28.3 gms = 1 oz.
16 ozs = 1 lb
1 lb = 0.453 kilogm
1 kilogm = 2.20 lbs

Cooking up herbal preparations is not difficult but there are certain tips that are worth knowing because they make the results a lot better and your life a whole lot easier. When using a blender, for instance, only do so with water-based liquids, not oils and waxes, otherwise too much air gets into the ingredients. Whenever a recipe specifies bringing something to the boil, you should do just that and then let the temperature drop back down again. Firstly this process makes sure the ingredients are sterile, and secondly it softens the water. Most water is rather hard, which spoils the emulsifying process and by boiling the water you soften it.

When beating a cream until it cools to get the right consistency, put the basin containing the cream in cold water. It speeds up the process and saves you getting wrist-ache. Another point worth mentioning is that when you mix oil from one pan with beeswax from another, always mix the oil *into* the wax, rather than vice versa. It's easier to clean an oily pan than one that has only contained wax.

We have not dealt with hair dyes but should you do so,

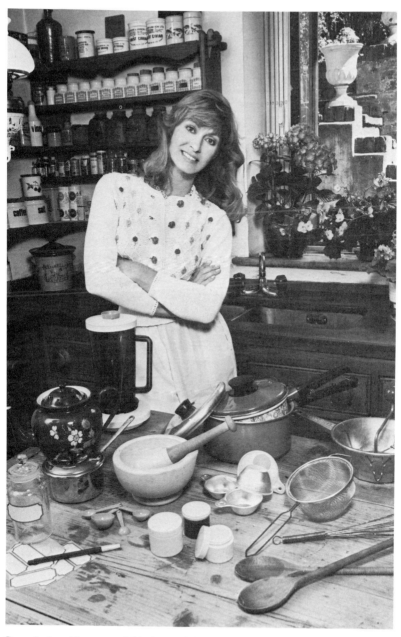

Suzy in her Hampstead kitchen with most of the equipment used for her cosmetic recipes. (Photographer—Mike Martin)

remember this cautionary tale. Suzy's sister Mary once dyed her mother's white hair a nice shade of brown by mixing together permanganate of potash with water. When she looked down at her own hands and arms, they were also a nice shade of brown, akin to the colour of a polished mahogany table, right up to the elbows. Mary was horrified and stayed away from school until the stain had worn off, which didn't help her education, but she has since learned that using a solution of sodium thiosulphate would have removed all the stains. The experience happily did not put her off hair dyes, and today she is a successful hairdresser in Derbyshire.

Our recipes do not call for preservatives because the only one available in the home is formalin, which is strong and is commonly used in funeral parlours, rather more suitable for creams for your late friends.

So keep most of the products you make in the refrigerator with the exception of some creams which become too hard. The average toner lasts about three weeks in the fridge and we have specified when ingredients are likely to spoil easily.

We have both had our own disasters. In Suzy's case she made an old Mrs Beeton remedy which stated that you mix 1 teaspoon of salt and 2 tablespoons of milk, rub gently over the skin and leave on overnight. Suzy recalls waking up the next morning under the distinct impression she'd been eating toast in bed! There were 'crumbs' everywhere and, what's more, the mixture was far too drying for her skin. When she got over the shock of that, she made up what she calls her Baby Cleansing Cream (see our recipes), which she's happy to report always worked well.

Pat's first attempt at making home remedies was after a particularly drying assault on her hair by the sun after making a commercial. In the hotel room, she beat two eggs into a little water and used the mixture as a shampoo and conditioner. It's been a staple of her beauty routine ever since as has the mixture of camomile and lemon, which she makes in a teapot with boiling water, allows to steep and

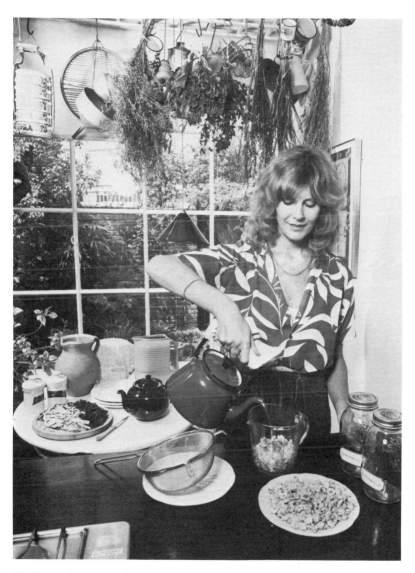

Pat in her kitchen making a camomile infusion for her hair, pouring boiling water onto camomile flowers. Next to the pyrex jug is a strainer for straining the infusion, when ready, into the screw-top jars to the right. Under the strainer is a plate to cover the jug whilst the flowers are steeping. On the table behind is nettle, waiting to be made into an infusion, quassia chips waiting to be simmered, and an assortment of suitable jugs. (Photographer—Mike Martin)

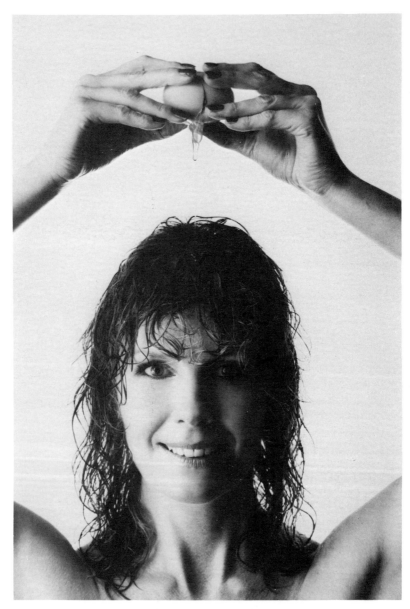

A little bit of artistic licence here. You actually need to beat two or three eggs together until fluffy and work them into wet hair. If your hair is very dry or damaged it really is a good, enriching treatment. (Photographer—Tim Simmons)

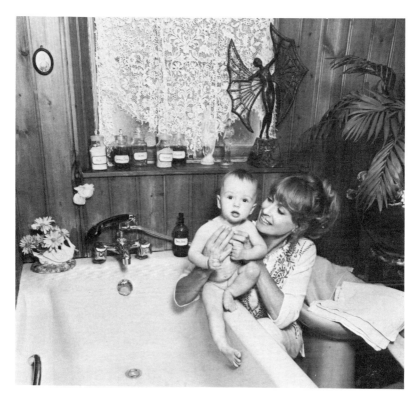

Bathfillers—a bundle of herbs, in a muslin handkerchief, with the string drawn tight, to hang under the running tap, milk, cinnamon sticks in almond oil, mixed herbs, oatmeal and vinegar. And a soft babybath of rosewater, with a few drops of our own coconut and protein shampoo—Suzy with daughter Elodie.
(Photographer—Mike Martin)

cool and pours over her hair as a final rinse. It's the ideal summer pick-up for fair hair that looks dull.

Allergies

It is always wise to test any recipes with a 'patch test' if you have sensitive skin or just want to be careful about what you put on your body. People can be allergic to almost anything, even water—so better safe than sorry. To do a 'patch test' place a small portion of cream, tonic or ingredient inside the crook of your elbow and cover with a clean plaster for 24 hours. If the skin does not become itchy or red during this time, you are not allergic to that particular substance.

It is also wise to boil all water used in recipes for 20 minutes, to use clean utensils, and to store your products in sterilised containers. Never keep home-made cosmetics for more than three weeks, even if stored in the fridge, and less where stated. Remember you are dealing with natural products which have no synthetic preservatives, and you have to be as careful with these as you would be with food.

None of our recipes is very complicated so we hope you will try them all. The masks are particularly rewarding for beginners because they rarely involve any cooking and can usually be mixed in minutes. All the treatments should improve your skin or hair but they should also raise your spirits, so above all, have fun.

6 The Herbs

The use of herbs in medicines, skin and hair care and cosmetics is, of course, as old as civilisation. Rediscovering old remedies has become increasingly popular of late, now that we have reached a point where sophisticated drugs, synthetics and chemicals seem to be a tidal wave that is engulfing us.

So, partly out of nostalgia for the simple and the natural and partly because the skin is our own, natural form of covering—and to treat it with natural products seems logical—herbs have again become important in skin and hair care.

So many commercial products are just too harsh—and expensive. As two women involved in a world where our appearance is important we both gravitated towards natural sources for our tonics and cleansers and hair treatments because we found ourselves reacting adversely to the unusual amount of punishment we imposed on our skin and hair.

Many herbs and useful plants can be grown in your windowbox or back garden, others you will find growing in hedgerows or even on wasteground if you know how to recognise them. And when you look into their backgrounds you will find almost all have Latin names which means they have been noted, tabulated and recognised for centuries. Some bear the word 'officinalis' in their name which indicates they were officially listed as being of medicinal value.

Storing and Drying Herbs

Our first choice would, of course, be a herb we have just plucked freshly from the soil but, since we live in the real world where seasons and geography limit our possibilities, it's worth learning the basics about drying herbs.

You can buy many of them packaged in neat jars in your local shops, but should you encounter difficulties we provide a list at the end of the book of specialist shops. If you have the time or the inclination, however, picking herbs on a sunny morning after the dew has evaporated from the ground is a lot more thrilling. On a practical level it also means that you control the quality and age of your products if you pick and dry them yourself.

Try not to handle the plants too much or you'll bruise the leaves. Herbs like thyme and rosemary, where the leaves are the part used, should be picked when the herb is just going to flower. In the case of camomile or lavender or any other plant whose flowers are used, wait until it is in full bloom before you pick it.

The easiest way to dry herbs is to find a warm, dry place out of the light and spread out the plants on a large piece of paper, making sure the air can circulate. You can also tie them into bunches (bearing name tags, otherwise you will forget what exactly is drying) and hang them upside down in any dark, warm place. It's a good idea to cover each bunch with newspaper to keep off the dust. Seed heads and pieces of bark can be dried simply by putting them in paper bags and hanging them up. If the weather is very damp and chilly and there's nowhere in your house that qualifies as a warm, dark place, then simply put your herbs in a rack in your oven on the *lowest* heat and let them dry slowly.

After they are dry, store the herbs in labelled, airtight jars or tins but try to avoid clear glass bottles or anything the light can penetrate. Little bottles of herbs may look very attractive but if it's efficacy you want, then a cool, dark and dry cupboard is your best bet.

Preparing Herbs

Remember to use enamel or non-metal pots and saucepans for herb preparation and whenever water is called for, always add distilled or mineral water as tap water can be hard and bad for your skin.

Infusions: Since we make so much reference to infusions in this book, we cannot emphasise enough that you make an infusion in the same way you'd make a pot of tea and, in the same way that you would never boil tea, do not boil the herbs. Instead you pour about a pint of boiling water over two tablespoons of dried leaves or flowers or four tablespoons of fresh leaves or flowers and let the mix steep in a warmed, covered pot for at least 15 minutes. Obviously, the longer the mixture stands, the stronger it will become, but three hours is about the time needed to reap the full benefit of the herb. After the infusion has steeped, the herbs will sink to the bottom of the pot and you can strain off the liquid ready for use as a hair rinse, toner, or whatever the herb is best used for.

Decoctions: This is just a matter of boiling the plant and is suitable for any recipe which requires that the roots, bark, seeds or chips of a plant are used. Simply simmer them steadily for about 30 minutes in a covered pan so you don't lose any of the fragrance or goodness. Allow to cool and strain.

Tinctures: This method is used for herbs that release their properties in alcohol but not in water. You have to pound one ounce of the herb until it's a powder and then add it to 12 fluid ounces of medicinal alcohol in a jar that has a tight-fitting lid. Let it stand for two weeks in bright sunlight or a warm place and remember to shake the jar every day. Before using, filter the tincture very thoroughly.

Essences: Take $\frac{1}{2}$ cup of crushed, fresh herbs or $\frac{1}{4}$ cup of crushed, dried herbs and add them to $\frac{3}{4}$ pint almond or sunflower oil. Mix in one tablespoon of white wine vinegar and pour the mixture into a jar or bottle with a tight lid. Shake well and then place the jar or bottle in a warm, sunny place and let it stand for three weeks. Strain well.

Now you are ready to select the herbs most suited to your own skin and hair and go to work with them. You can use the infusions neat or you can add them to recipes in place of distilled water or rosewater. Simple oils can be replaced by essences of herbs. The idea is that you should experiment until you find which methods and herbs work best for you, then you can create your own herbal signature.

Meadow and Woodland Herbs

Lady's Mantle (*Alchemilla vulgaris*). Pat first found this little perennial with yellow-green flowers when she was taking a walk in the dales of Yorkshire. She picked what she thought was a wild flower and then found it pictured and listed in an encyclopaedia of herbs as being useful for sensitive skin as a toner. It was very popular in the sixteenth and seventeenth centuries when herbalists called it the 'wound' herb because it was good for drying up sores. Use the kidney-shaped leaves.

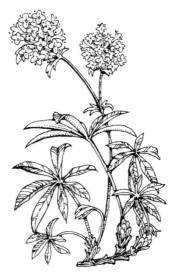

Lady's Mantle

Elder (*Sambucus nigra*). Cream-coloured flowers and black berries mark out this little tree which is a repository of folklore. Witches were afraid of the elder tree because the

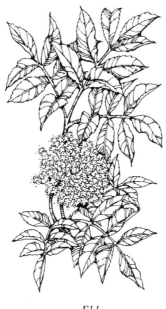

Elder

Cross of Calvary was reputedly hewn out of elder. The elder
is also supposed to ward off evil influences and a twig of it,
carried in the pocket, is said to be a cure against rheumatism.
All that's as may be, but we use it in skin tonics for a slight
astringent effect which reduces enlarged pores. The elder
flowers in June should be collected and used fresh but you
can also salt the flowers (just add 10% common salt) to
'pickle' or preserve the blossoms. Elder leaves are used to
make 'oil of swallows' (one part crushed elder leaves to three
parts linseed oil) which horsemen use to give the coats of
their animals a wonderful shine. We have tried using a little
on the ends of our hair and it does work. Pat's grandmother,
a true Victorian, used to swear by elderflower water to keep
her skin pale and blemish-free.

Nettles (*Urtica dioica*). Yes, the common stinging
nettle has its uses. Found in wasteland, in cottage gardens,
meadows and woodland areas it has quite a history. The
Romans are said to have found our English climate a little

chilly and so they kept warm by rubbing nettles on their bare skin to give themselves a burning sensation! We would never advocate this method of fuel economy but as a stimulating, anti-dandruff hair rinse, the nettle is very effective. The whole plant should be cut off just above the root before it flowers in late May or early June and, if you find the smell of nettles a little overwhelming when making your rinse, add a few drops of oil of lavender. Nettle rinse is also said to restore colour to greying hair and add gloss to hair that has gone dull from illness.

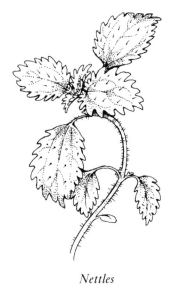

Nettles

Juniper (*Juniperis communis*). This shrub grows more successfully in Europe, particularly Hungary, than it does in Britain although it can still be found in Wiltshire, on chalky, southern exposures and in the central highlands of Scotland. The juniper produces berries that take up to three years to ripen to the dark, blue colour that they should be when harvested. The best known use of these berries is as the prime ingredient in gin but oil of juniper is used throughout Europe as a curative for the digestive system. Juniper berries are reputed to be an effective cure against alopecia, if used regularly. We use juniper in our commercial hair conditioner, along with birch, burdock, camomile and marigold.

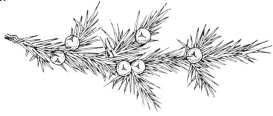

Juniper

Red Clover (*Trifolium pratense*). Clover is a corruption of the word 'clava' or club, as portrayed in a pack of playing cards. And we all know what luck has apportioned us if we find a four-leaf clover. Most of us, however, will have to be satisfied with three-leaf clover and this will do very nicely as a gentle skin cleansing wash after the flowers have been made into an infusion.

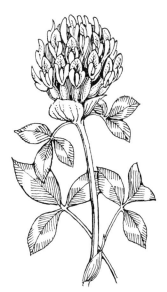

Red Clover

Camomile (*Authemis nobilis*). Wild camomile is the type used in natural beauty products and it is the small, daisy-like flowers that are so valuable in infusions for skin and hair. Pat swears by them, to give lights to her hair. For centuries this type of camomile has been made into a tea and used as a nerve sedative and even a soporific. The whole plant is greyish green and covered in down and you will find it growing on dry commons and in sandy soil.

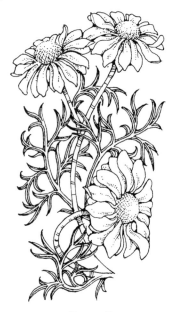

Camomile

Eyebright (*Euphrasia officinalis*). Since the Middle Ages, eyebright has been used as an eye lotion to counter tiredness and red eyes. This elegant little plant flowers in late summer and is identifiable by its many small, white or purple flowers variegated with yellow. Eyebright is part of the foxglove family of plants and more than 200 species grow in the British Isles in chalky soil, particularly close to the sea. Its Latin name is actually derived from the Greek and means 'to see well' and the entire plant, picked when in full flower, can make a soothing eye lotion.

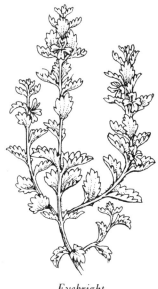

Eyebright

Comfrey (Symphytum officinale). Bell-shaped flowers
that can be blue, pink, purple or even cream mark out this
useful herb which grows in watermeadows and by river
banks. Traditionally comfrey was grown in the herb gardens
of monasteries where the monks used to call it 'knitbone'
because it was considered helpful for healing broken bones,
sprains, bruises and even backache. As a little girl, Pat would
have her sprains and bruises wrapped in bandages that had

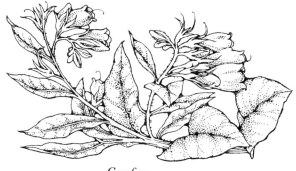

Comfrey

been immersed in comfrey juice. Today we both find comfrey invaluable as a soothing skin and hair infusion, we add it to our commercial strawberry shampoo, and we have been told that taking a long bath in comfrey is very rejuvenating for the skin. Search out the plant and pick its leaves during the summer months and use these for your infusions.

Burdock (Arcticum lappa). This herb grows wild in abundance and the largest of the species, the great burdock, is a familiar sight by roadsides with its rhubarb-like leaves which are white underneath. Burdock is called by many local names including Love Leaves and Beggar's Buttons but because of its shape it is more often called Gipsy's Rhubarb. The root and the seeds of the plant are used to make a cooling, soothing lotion and burdock, when mixed with the white of an egg, is a help in healing burns.

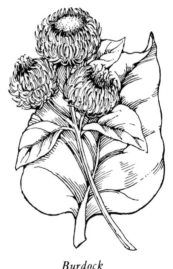

Burdock

Valerian (Cypripedium pubescens). Three types of this plant grow in England. Pat first found the plant with its pink flowers growing by the river in the Vale of Blackmoor, and it

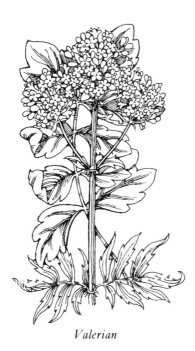

Valerian

certainly likes watery places. Folklore has it that the herb was
hung up by the door of the house to bring peace to the home
and prevent marital bickering and, although we cannot attest
to its efficacy in that area, we do know it helps the skin's
water balance, thus counteracting drying, and has a relaxing
effect if used in the bath.

Birch (*Betula alba*). 'The Lady of the Woods'
Coleridge called this elegant, silver tree of which the bark
and the leaves have many uses. The birch is slender and
hardy and grows high on mountains, in woodlands and in
country gardens and city parks. The bark, when distilled,
yields birch tar oil which is used as a soothing ointment for
skin problems like eczema and, when mixed with other oils,
works as an insect repellent. The American Indian tribes
used birch to make a tea to counter rheumatism and today
we have found birch is a good scalp cleanser and stimulates
hair growth.

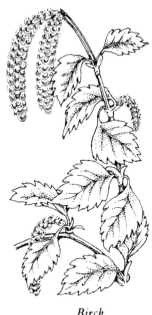

Birch

Cottage Garden Herbs

Rosemary (Rosmarinus officinalis). This herb became symbolic as an emblem of fidelity for lovers and so it became traditional for a young bride to wear rosemary on her wedding day. Anyone who has visited the Mediterranean will have found themselves in fields of sweet-smelling rosemary and it is also common in Britain where it has been cultivated in herb gardens for centuries. This perennial shrub has grey-green, needle-like leaves and pale blue flowers which bloom erratically throughout the summer months. Rosemary is fragrant, easily dried and well-known as beneficial to the hair and scalp. You can use fresh or dried leaves for a mild rinse or make a stronger infusion as a lotion which can be rubbed into the scalp to help counteract dandruff and to aid hair health and growth. Suzy keeps a mixture of rosemary and lavender in a jar in her bathroom and throws a handful in the running water for an aromatic bath.

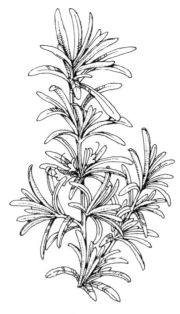

Rosemary

Parsley (*Carum petroselinum*). For the Ancient Greeks, parsley was used in the same way as laurel leaves, to crown the victors of athletic events and as wreaths for the dead. Today parsley is most common as a decoration on restaurant plates, but it is full of Vitamin C and should be eaten or

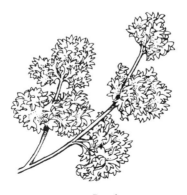

Parsley

turned into an infusion which is particularly good for troubled, blemished skin. Parsley is also a breath freshener. You will find this familiar plant growing in moist shady places. Try picking the entire herb fresh and using it immediately.

Lavender (*Lavandula vera*). The word itself is derived from the Latin 'lavo' to wash because Romans used lavender to scent their bath water. To this day, lavender is one of the most fragrant of herbs and in England one of the easiest to find. There are, of course, many varieties but all have beautifully scented flowers and leaves that flower in July. English lavender is much more aromatic than the French and so the oil fetches ten times the price. The principal lavender areas are in Surrey, Suffolk and Kent and the flowers should be in full bloom when harvested. Remember to pick your lavender early in the morning or at dusk and *never* on a rainy day. Dried lavender flowers are wonderful in bags when used to perfume linen and the scent does help repel moths. Oil of

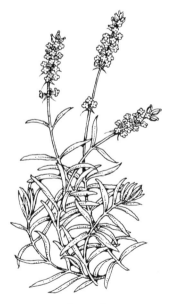

Lavender

lavender, when applied to freshly brushed hair, helps sort out
the knots and tangles and is good for the scalp. Suzy has
three lavender bushes growing in her garden. She says they
are easy to cultivate and, besides the smell, look beautiful
among the other flowers.

Marigold (*Calendula officinalis*). Marigolds grow in
cultivated English gardens and also wild in the vineyards of
Europe, although they are believed to have originated in
India. Marigolds start flowering in June and continue until
the frost kills them. Originally, marigolds were used as

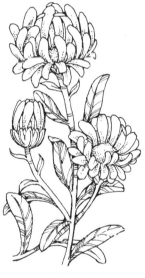

Marigold

healing plants for wounds. Today we use them in tincture
form rubbed into the scalp to help hair growth, and also we
soak the petals in oil and rub them on the skin as a
complexion healer.

Lemon Balm (*Melissa officinalis*). This two-to-three
feet high bush has a delightful fragrance that attracts bees to
its lemon-scented leaves. The leaves are pale green and heart-

shaped with small, whitish flowers during summer. In the
Middle Ages lemon balm was strewn over the rushes that
covered the dirty floors to impart a good smell to the
houses. These days its chief use is as a bath-time herb or to
add to a pot-pourri or a herbal sleeping pillow because of its
delicate scent. Cut the stems of the bush at the end of the
summer, tie into bunches and after drying add to your bath
in little muslin bags.

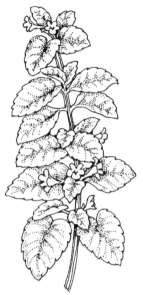

Lemon Balm

Cowslip (*Primula veris*). The plant, which is
consecrated to St Peter, is said to represent safety and
security. It is typical of the English countryside and the
flowers can be used to make cowslip wine, which is said to
be soothing for nervous complaints, and these days cowslip
flowers are made into infusions which work as gentle skin
cleansers. The leaves are similar to those of a primrose and
the plant has long stalks which are crowned by flowers.
These have a very distinctive and fresh fragrance and are
delightful if used fresh during the summer months.

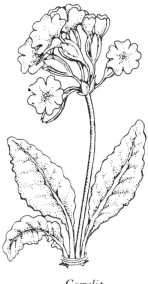

Cowslip

Thyme (*Thymus vulgaris*). This beautifully scented perennial has tiny, dark leaves and grows as a bush. Thyme should be picked during its July flowering time and the herb

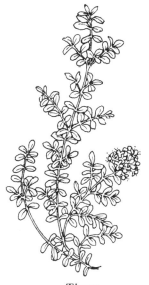

Thyme

responds very well to drying, losing little of its properties. Wild thyme resembles the cultivated variety but has less of a scent although it is very good in tonic form for reducing large pores when used as an infusion or dried and pounded into a cream. Thyme has properties that stimulate the peripheral circulation of the skin and it works as a toner and helps clear up spots.

Yarrow (*Achillea millefolium*). From June to September, little daisy-like flowers bloom on stalks that are covered in silky hairs. In old times soldiers used to dress wounds with the herb, hence yarrow used to be known as Soldiers Wound Wort. The whole plant can be culled during the month of August when it is in flower and made into decoctions or infusions which are used as tonics and fresheners, particularly freshening for oily or greasy skin.

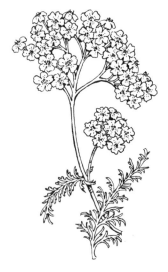

Yarrow

Tansy (*Tanacetum vulgare*). Otherwise known as Buttons, tansy has large, dull yellow flowers with feathery leaves that bloom in clusters in late summer. Wild tansy has a stronger scent than the garden tansy but both thrive in almost any type of soil. The leaves have been used for centuries for dealing with problems as divergent as hysteria and kidney weakness. Used externally, tansy has long been considered beneficial to skin eruptions and, due to its properties when made into a tonic, has been passed on to us as a way of fading freckles.

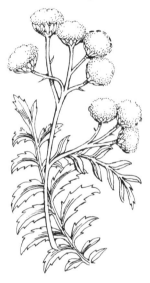

Tansy

Mint (*Mentha*). There are several kinds of mint but the plant known generally as mint and used in cooking is spearmint. This fragrant, hardy herb originated in the East and was brought to our country by the Romans and has many delightful uses. Balm mint opens the pores and stimulates the skin which is why we chose it as a base for the cleanser we sell. Mint has an astringent effect on enlarged pores, helping reduce and tighten them. Pick your mint for drying when the flowers are in bud; you can either dry the entire plant or take the leaves off the stalks and dry them alone.

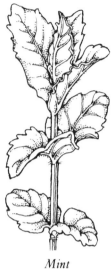

Mint

Fennel (*Foeniculum vulgare*). This perennial herb grows in Devon and Cornwall, often in a semi-wild state and in chalky spots in Wales and Kent. It has feathery leaves and little yellow flowers but it is the leaves, roots and seeds which are used for medicinal and cosmetic purposes. The plant has

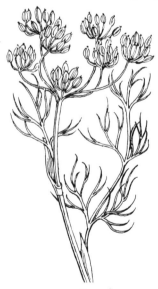

Fennel

a delicate, aniseed scent which is stronger in the seeds when dried than in the leaves. Fennel has long been used to counter wrinkles and its culinary uses are legendary.

Some Exotic Herbs and Plants

Peruvian Bark (*Cinchona officinalis*). The inhabitants of Peru passed on the bark of the quinine tree, otherwise known as Peruvian Bark, to the Spanish conquerors who brought it back to Europe. The Jesuits used it in a powdered form for those suffering from fever and malaria. The bark comes from evergreen trees which bear fragrant flowers of crimson and dark rose. We don't suggest you try to grow this plant because it thrives in the mountainous regions of places like Java. But you can buy the dried stem bark in certain shops in England (see list at end of book) and make a decoction which promotes hair growth and is good as a final rinse.

Papaya, otherwise known as Pawpaw (*Papaya vulgaris*). When Suzy was filming in Hawaii, she first encountered this rich fruit which is also known as Melon Tree. Large spreading leaves mark out the tree and at the base of these leaves you will find the fruit which varies in colour from a pale, greenish-yellow to a deep, ripe orange. A white powder is made from the juices of the papaya, for medicinal purposes. But the makeup artist on Suzy's film advised her to try rubbing the flesh of a ripe papaya fruit directly onto her face as a toning mask.

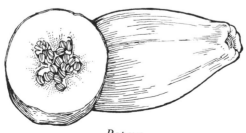

Papaya

Ginseng (*Panax quinquefolium*). The Chinese considered ginseng a panacea for almost any disease or illness so the Emperors monopolised the rights to harvest the roots and, indeed, wars were fought over them. There are different types of ginseng which grow in both the East and the United States. Red Korean ginseng is the most prized and expensive

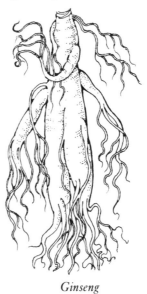

Ginseng

variety. When Pat was travelling in Thailand and Malaysia, she was introduced to ginseng by some local people who gave her the ash-coloured powder to take against a bad cold she had contracted. They also told her that a little ginseng, taken daily, does wonders for the skin and one's general health. You can buy the powdered root or take ginseng tablets.

Aloe (*Aloe vera*). There are several types of aloe, all of which are succulent plants belonging to the lily family with fleshy leaves and fibrous, strong roots. It grows in the tropics, where it flowers almost all year long. Suzy found it when she was in the West Indies and, again, came across it in Hawaii. When she heard that the plant was known as a healer of sunburns and would conserve a suntan, she started by trying to pound the leaves into a pulp and put the resulting thick juice on her skin. Aloe Vera is not available in many countries so it's difficult to make up your own aloe creams. However, we now import Aloe Vera for our commercial products and have incorporated it in a shampoo, a moisturiser which also has Vitamin E in it, and a body lotion which really does help prolong a tan.

Quassia (Picraena excelsa). This tree, otherwise known as Bitter Ash, grows in Jamaica, Antigua and St Vincent and we both encountered it for the first time in Jamaica. The trees grow to about 60 feet tall and, although they have no odour, the taste of the bark is very bitter. The wood is generally sold in small chips and boiled up to make a tonic for the digestion. If made into a decoction, the quassia chips can be mixed with camomile to make a rinse to lighten fair hair.

Jojoba (pronounced Hohoba). This plant grows in Mexico and the Southern USA and produces a bean from which oil is extracted. It is, in our view, quite remarkable in that all other known vegetable oils are not absorbed into the skin whereas Jojoba is. The result of this is that while most cosmetic companies have used synthetic esters in their

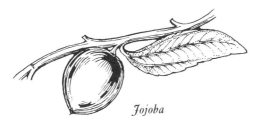

Jojoba

products, in our search for natural ingredients we were introduced to this oil which we immediately had made into a moisturising cream, the first of its type in England. Jojoba is not generally available but it is now being widely grown commercially and should be in selected shops in the near future.

7 Recipes for Face, Hair and Skin

Cleansers

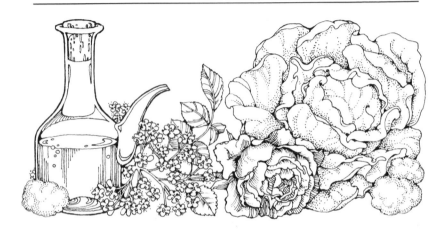

If there is one basic beauty secret that any model or actress will tell you, it's never to go to bed without cleaning your face. However tired you may feel, whatever the hour or the temptations, spend a few minutes removing the day's grime, grease and makeup.

You cannot look good the next day if you don't cleanse properly the night before because your skin will become dull and lifeless and blackheads will result from the clogged pores. Even worse, if you regularly go to bed without cleansing, your skin will actually coarsen and age.

The controversy of soap and water versus cleansing cream is one that has raged for a long while. Soap and water do remove grime but they can't lift out the waxy base that exists in most makeups. Soap is generally very drying and those soaps that claim to be PH balanced and therefore supposedly maintain the acid-alkaline balance simply do not live up to their reputations, in our experience.

So we would suggest a simple cleansing routine of a cream or milk followed by a toner or refresher. The cleansing cream will remove the grime and old makeup and by gently massaging the skin as you rub off the cream, you'll stimulate the circulation of the blood bringing oxygen to the surface which will feed your skin. Massage with either your fingertips or a complexion brush, though we recommend you remove the cream with tissues rather than a face flannel, as the latter often harbours grease and is difficult to wash out properly.

Don't forget to tissue off the cream with an upward movement. Dragging the skin downwards just encourages lines and wrinkles.

Old-Fashioned Lettuce Cleanser

This is one of the simplest cleansers known to woman. Wash a head of lettuce, put it in a non-aluminium saucepan and cover with boiling water. Put on a lid and simmer for an hour. Strain the liquid into a jar and add a few drops of tincture of benzoin. Keep in the fridge and use when chilled.

Elderflower Cleansing Milk

This is another easy recipe and delightfully fragrant. Simmer six tbsps of elderflower blossoms in $\frac{1}{2}$ pint of milk for 30 minutes or until the blossoms are soft. Take it off the heat, cover and leave for three hours. Strain the scented milk, bottle it and refrigerate. Night and morning dip a cotton wool pad in the sweet-smelling mixture, and, with upward strokes, clean the face.

When Suzy's skin was left particularly parched by a film she made in the sun, the professional makeup man gave her a tip to try making up her own cleanser from cocoa butter which is exceptionally nutritious:

Cocoa Butter Cleanser
3 ozs cocoa butter
1 oz almond oil
2 ozs rosewater

Slowly melt the cocoa butter over a low heat while in another saucepan warm the almond oil. Gradually, drop by drop, add the warmed oil and the rosewater to the cocoa butter, beating all the time. Remove from heat and continue beating until quite smooth. Leave to cool.

Oatmeal Cleanser (for oily skin)

2 tbsps oatmeal (not instant or 1-minute, you don't want a porridge)
2 ozs glycerine
2 ozs mineral oil

Heat the glycerine and mineral oil together and beat. Take off the heat. When cool add the oatmeal. Use with a circular washing motion to benefit from the gently abrasive action.

Strawberry Cleansing Cream

6 tbsps petroleum jelly
1 tbsp strained fresh strawberry juice
Pinch of borax

Melt the petroleum jelly over a very low heat, dissolve the borax into the strawberry juice and beat thoroughly into the melted petroleum jelly until the consistency is creamy and the mixture has cooled. Keep in the fridge.

If you love the scent of strawberries and can't be bothered to make the simple cream above, just cut fresh strawberries in half and pulp them on your face. The strawberries act as a mild astringent and will help get rid of any oiliness and encourage circulation. They are also a skin-whitener.

Rose Petal Cleanser

4 tbsps almond oil
3 tbsps rosewater
1 oz dried rose petals
$\frac{3}{4}$ oz beeswax

This formula of oil, wax and water has been used for centuries to cleanse and soften the skin. Soak the rose petals in the rosewater for three days, then strain. In a pudding basin standing in a large saucepan of boiling water put the oil and the wax and wait until the wax dissolves. Remove from the heat. Add strained rosewater, drop by drop, beating all the time. Keep beating until cool, then store in your fridge.

Cucumber Cleansing Cream

3 tsps beeswax
3 tsps almond oil
3 tsps olive oil
3 tsps sunflower oil
4 tsps cucumber juice (made from $\frac{1}{4}$ cucumber which
    has been mashed and strained or put in a blender)
$\frac{1}{2}$ tsp borax

Melt the oils and wax in an enamel pan set in a larger pan full of hot water. In a separate bowl warm the cucumber juice and borax and add that mixture drop by drop into the oil, stirring constantly. Remove from the heat and beat until cool. Keep in fridge.

Fast Fruit Cleanser

6 tbsps coconut oil
2 tbsps strained fruit juice (strawberry, lemon,
    watermelon or you can even use a vegetable like
    carrots)
$\frac{1}{4}$ tsp borax

Melt the oil over a low heat. Dissolve the borax in the warmed fruit juice and then beat into the oil until cool. This fruit cleanser is quick, simple and wonderful to use but remember to keep it in the fridge. It's nicer to use cold and it will last much longer. Keep for approx. one week.

Baby Cleansing Cream

3 tbsps baby oil
4 tsps beeswax
1 tbsp witch hazel
1 tbsp water
1 tbsp almond oil
$\frac{1}{4}$ tsp borax
(optional: a few drops of perfume or an essential oil
    such as lemon)

Melt the beeswax and oils in a pudding basin standing in a large saucepan of boiling water. Dissolve the borax in warmed witch hazel and water (here add perfume or light and fresh lemon essential oil, if you wish). Pour this slowly into the oil and wax mixture, beating all the time until cool. Again, once you have put it into a jar or pot, keep it refrigerated.

Dry Skin Cleanser

Yolk of one egg
2 tsps glycerine

Beat the glycerine into the egg yolk and apply to the face with fingertips. Leave until it dries, then wash off with warm water. Keep any leftovers in the fridge for another time.

Tonics

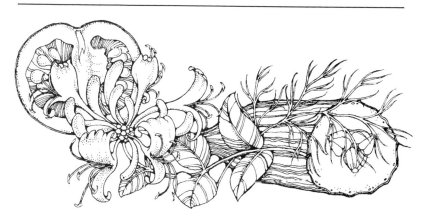

Tonics work in two ways. They refresh the skin and make you feel good but they also finish the work begun by cleansing creams and lotions by removing the last vestiges of grease from the face and neck. Plain, old-fashioned cold water splashed on the face tightens the pores and makes you feel cooler. After you've cooked a meal, any vegetable water, strained and refrigerated, has the same effect and is additionally beneficial because it puts vitamins directly onto the skin. And it certainly needs no special effort to prepare. Simple mixes of rosewater, witch hazel (and drops of glycerine, if your skin is very dry) work perfectly well and don't dry out the precious moisture in your skin.

You will see that our own products are not listed as being for any particular skin type because, in our experience, all skin types benefit from *mild stimulation*. However, if we feel specific homemade recipes benefit oily skins more than dry, or vice versa, we will say so. But a word of caution. Use anything that is harsh or strong rarely and very sparingly.

A harsh astringent applied to problem skin only stimulates the glands to produce more toxins. The body over-compensates and produces more sweat and therefore more problems. In our experience, problem skins more than any other need a mild tonic, but used more often, say three or four times a day. Our Cool Cucumber Toner is ideal for this, if you don't want to make your own.

Remember when you're applying tonics that you are not actually putting the lotion *on* your skin, you are wiping your face clean with it. Use upward strokes and don't rub too hard. Both of us have learned to use refreshing toners throughout the day when we've been working under harsh lights. Professional makeup artists on films and commercials gently wipe the centre panel of the face—forehead, nose, crease lines and chin—when the makeup looks jaded and then reapply a thin layer of fresh makeup over the top. This prevents makeup from caking and getting that 'lived-in' look.

You can buy mineral water sprays that help you feel fresh, are good for removing just surface grime and leave you ready to reapply any new makeup you want to your skin. A professional's trick is to use these sprays for setting the makeup. Once an actress has her face done and is ready for filming, the makeup man will gently spray her face with a very fine mist from a mineral water spray, thus softening the look.

At least once a week steam your skin to open the pores before you clean it. Do this by covering your head with a towel over a large bowl of boiling water for ten minutes, but be careful not to put your face too near—about a foot away is perfect. Otherwise you could get broken veins or too dry skin. Try putting fennel in the water. It's good against wrinkles and has a delicious smell. But remember to be gentle with your skin, stroking your tonic or freshener on gently afterwards.

Some of the earliest recipes for fresheners and tonics are made from rosewater. You can buy it in just about every chemist shop but you can also make your own by taking a couple of handfuls of sweet-smelling rose petals, putting them in a jar and covering them with a pint of hot water and a handful of sugar. Put a lid over the mixture and shake it hard. Then let it stand for a couple of hours, shake again and strain. Store it in your fridge or in a cool place.

Suzy's mother-in-law has made up her own basic tonic for many years:

Rosemary's Rosewater Freshener

In proportion, mix $\frac{2}{3}$ of rosewater (your homemade kind, as above, is cheaper), with $\frac{1}{3}$ of witch hazel and then slowly add a few drops of glycerine. Mix well, keep cool and shake before using.

Remember to make any preparation in small amounts and often, rather than in huge pots. Keep it cool in the fridge and it should last you three weeks or more. But, again, little and often is undoubtedly the secret here.

Apple Freshener

This is another very simple recipe. Just take 1 oz apple vinegar, 2 ozs witch hazel, shake together and cool. (You'll see that witch hazel is a regular feature of many fresheners and the reason for this is that it has been known for centuries for its healing properties. It seems to reduce any puffiness or swelling and works as a mild antiseptic.)

Cucumber Toner—for Open Pores

This is one of our favourites, as it leaves the skin feeling cool and not at all dry. After being subjected to all kinds of cosmetics and the often adverse conditions of a studio or location, we both have occasionally found ourselves with a few open pores. This freshener gently, very gently, tightens the skin and leaves it with a fresh, tangy, clean feeling.

$1\frac{1}{2}$ tsps glycerine
$1\frac{1}{2}$ ozs alcohol or eau de cologne
4 ozs witch hazel
2 ozs cucumber juice
$\frac{1}{4}$ tsp tincture of benzoin

Squeeze or put in a blender a quarter of a cucumber, including the skin, and strain. Add all the other ingredients, put them in a pretty old bottle and shake well. Keep this mix in the fridge, but remember, it doesn't last long because it's very perishable, so use immediately.

Simple Cucumber Toner

This can be used anytime but it is particularly nice on a hot day. Put a quarter of a cucumber in a blender, strain off the juice and add the same amount of witch hazel to the liquid you have from the cucumber. Cool and, once again, put in the fridge, because although cucumber has lovely cooling properties, it goes off very quickly.

Lettuce Tonic

$\frac{1}{4}$ head of lettuce (you can substitute carrots or celery)
1 glass water
$\frac{1}{2}$ tsp tincture of benzoin

Chop the lettuce into small pieces and, with the glass of cold water, put in a blender at a high speed. Strain through a fine sieve or a nylon stocking and put the liquid in the refrigerator for one day. Strain twice more and add the tincture of benzoin, shake vigorously and use—but you might want to wait until the deep chill has gone off it.

Tomato Tonic

2 tbsps whey of milk
Sieved juice of a fresh tomato

Shake together in a bottle or in a blender until well mixed, apply to the face with cotton wool. Remove the remains after ten minutes with warm water, then splash with cold.

Mint and Parsley Tonic

$\frac{1}{4}$ cup chopped parsley
1 tbsp dried mint

Pour a cup of boiling water over the ingredients. Cover and leave for an hour. Strain into a container and use after cleaning your face. Don't keep this mix more than three days, it doesn't last long.

Tonic for Dry Skin

$\frac{1}{4}$ cup milk of magnesia
4 tbsps oil of avocado
4 tbsps rosewater
1 tsp borax
$\frac{1}{4}$ tsp oil of orange (an essential oil and optional in this recipe)

Beat together the milk of magnesia and the avocado oil. Slowly dissolve the borax in the rosewater which has been warmed. Mix well and add the orange oil, if you plan to use it. Then beat this mixture with the milk and the oil until you have a rich liquid. Keep cool.

Tonic for Greasy Skin

$\frac{1}{4}$ cup white wine vinegar
$\frac{1}{2}$ cup water
1 tsp cream of tartar

Mix the cream of tartar with water in a bowl or a blender until the two ingredients are well blended. Then add the vinegar and shake well. Each time you use it, shake well again. Remove after ten minutes with warm water and splash with cold.

Lavender Skin Tonic

Pat's grandmother used to clean her face with this mixture and, if her complexion was anything to go by, it works! You can replace the lavender with marigold, dandelion or honeysuckle if you prefer.

Pour about half a pint of boiling water over a handful

of lavender in a small saucepan, cover and simmer very gently for fifteen minutes. Then let the mixture stand for an hour, strain and cool and it's ready to use. Lavender has a particularly soothing effect, as well as smelling wonderful. Dandelions are said to help the 'dead' look that dark skin can get and honeysuckle, as well as being delightfully aromatic, has healing properties.

As you have seen, skin fresheners are easy to make and very pleasant to use. Vinegar appears in a great many traditional recipes because the skin has an acid mantle and the acidic quality in vinegar restores this mantle. Suzy, who has very sensitive skin, always keeps a large bottle of vinegar (any type from the poshest to the lowliest, it doesn't matter) in her bathroom and adds it to her bathwater and final hair rinse. It gets rid of that itchy feeling and she has found that continual use has eliminated the fine rash she would sometimes get on her neck and shoulders. Always dilute the vinegar thoroughly, one part to ten parts of water.

Masks

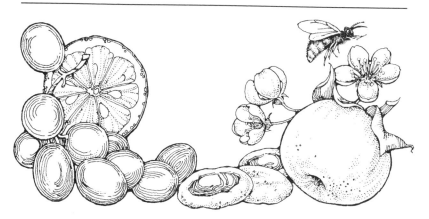

There are a lot of good reasons for using a mask regularly but the best we know are that masks are both simple and fun to make and very beneficial to your skin. Most of the ingredients are probably already in your kitchen.

Masks perform many valuable functions for us, they can tighten the skin, lighten the colour, get rid of the surface accumulation of dead cells and moisturise. But all masks have one basic function in common: they deep cleanse, lift out impurities, soften and leave the skin feeling wonderfully fresh and alive.

Try using a different mask every week, or a favourite regularly, and you will soon notice the difference in your complexion. Too many people have a cleansing routine which works well for every day, but they don't bother to luxuriate once a week, thus missing the physical and emotional benefits which are well worth the effort involved.

First, make sure that, once you've made the mask of your choice, you have enough time to let it sit on your face for 15 or 20 minutes. Your hair should be tied back out of the way, all wisps should be clinched with a hair band or towel and you should be wearing a dressing gown or bathtowel, in case the stuff drips.

It's important to relax after applying a mask, for not only will your skin get the chance to benefit properly from the ingredients of the mask but the opportunity to lie down and put your feet up will do you almost as much good as the mask itself.

Having prepared the mask you plan to use and got yourself ready and preferably alone—no one would *choose* to be seen with their hair scraped back and a lot of goo on their face—fill a basin with hot water, throw in a handful of scented herbs of your choice and steam your face with a towel over your head and covering the bowl or basin. This process opens up all the pores, loosens any blackheads so that you can easily remove them with clean tissues and improves circulation while deep cleaning the skin.

Remember not to get too close to the hot water, otherwise you could end up with broken veins, and only steam your face for about ten minutes. The herbs you add can be useful as well as smelling good—camomile is soothing, fennel is good for wrinkles, comfrey is healing, mint and sage are noted for being good pore openers.

For dry skin mix a pinch of each of the following together: comfrey leaf, comfrey root, camomile flowers, cloverheads, pansy and kelp. Place them all in a covered pot full of water and bring to the boil. Simmer for five minutes then remove from the heat and steam your face as usual. For oily skin use the following herbs in the same way: comfrey leaf, lavender flowers, lemon peel, mint (preferably peppermint), parsley and strawberry leaves.

After the steaming process, wipe your face with a clean tissue.

This is the time to start applying the mask itself, which should be a cooling, fragrant, pleasant sensation that helps you relax for those vital 15–20 minutes. We have found that putting the mask on with a man's shaving brush is a good way to control the amount used and best for applying the thicker masks. But your fingers are just as good if you don't have a clean shaving brush handy. Never apply a mask to an open wound and never put it around the eyes.

On the eyes place two pads of cotton wool moistened with cold water or one of your mild tonics. These pads shut out the light and soothe the eyes. Two squeezed, used tea bags is another good idea.

A nice tip that Suzy picked up from an Italian actress on one film set was to put honey on the delicate eye area while the mask is on the rest of the face. Apart from being a natural moisturiser, honey is very healing, helps to soften sensitive skin and is ideally nourishing used in this way.

If you have dark circles under your eyes, try putting dried figs over the area as you rest and while the mask goes to work. Figs are full of protein and are effective in banishing those heavy shadows.

Remove masks by washing your face with warm or tepid water until all traces of the mask have vanished, then splash with cold water, unless otherwise directed.

Masks sometimes sound like a lot of bother but, providing you have 20 minutes to yourself, it is time well spent. All the little impurities that lodge in the skin are coaxed up to the surface by the drawing power in the masks, and regular, weekly use can banish these problems forever. Don't forget that your face, unlike the rest of your body, is exposed not just to wind and rain and sun but also to pollution and grime and, of course, to cosmetics. Your face deserves a little extra care and none of the recipes we have tried have turned out to be complicated. Sometimes they can be messy, but they work, and there is nothing like a mask to make you feel pampered.

Grape, Yoghurt and Honey Basic Mask

This is soothing, penetrating, moisturising and, what's more, a great recipe to begin with because you cannot go wrong. All you need are equal parts of honey and plain yoghurt, with a handful of mashed grapes added. Mix them together and apply to your clean, freshly-steamed face. The grapes are particularly beneficial to sun-dried skin because the acidity in the fruit helps to replace the skin's acid mantle.

Yoghurt is particularly useful for anyone with a greasy skin and you can add a spoonful of it to almost any of the following recipes; we think you'll find it works particularly well when mixed with fruit. Bear in mind that yoghurt is also a mild bleach so it's good for any winter-dingy oily skin. One of the joys of a yoghurt and fruit mask is that it's as good to eat as it is to put on your face. So eat up any excess!

Beetroot Anti-Wrinkle Mask

If you suffer from fine lines and wrinkles, grate a raw beetroot with enough fresh thick cream to make a paste. Apply this all over a clean skin. Again, this mask is simplicity itself and very nourishing for dried and tired skins.

Apricot and Almond Healing Mask

Dried apricots are full of Vitamin A and this mask is wonderful for skin that needs healing and replenishing.

6 dried apricots, soaked overnight
1 tsp almond oil
1 tsp honey
$\frac{1}{2}$ tsp witch hazel

Mash the apricots, add the other ingredients to the fruity purée, and it's ready to use.

Almond, Cucumber and Lemon Scrub (for oily skin)

3 tbsps almonds
$\frac{1}{2}$ fresh cucumber
Juice of $\frac{1}{2}$ lemon

Pulverise the almonds in a blender until very fine, wash the cucumber and put in a blender, skin and all. Mix the two ingredients evenly together and slowly add the lemon juice until you have a paste. When removing the mask, after about 15–20 minutes, use warm water applied with a circular washing movement so the abrasive action removes any dead cells. Splash your face with cold water.

Grapefruit and Oat Scrub (for oily skin)

3–4 tbsps oatmeal
Juice of one grapefruit

Mash the oatmeal, or blend until fine, then slowly add the grapefruit juice until a paste is formed. This works in the same way as Almond Cucumber and Lemon Scrub and should be removed in the same way, thus getting the full benefit of the 'abrasiveness' of the oatmeal.

Strawberry Mask (for oily skin)

2 ozs fuller's earth
4 large fresh strawberries

Mash and strain the strawberries and add gradually to the fuller's earth until a paste is formed, like a 'mud pack'. The fuller's earth is noted for its pulling power and drying properties and the strawberries work as an astringent.

Egg and Lemon Mask (for oily skin)

1 egg white
Juice of one lemon

Whip up the egg white until really frothy then beat in the lemon juice. The egg white works as a skin tightener while the lemon juice has astringent and bleaching qualities. This particular mask is very thin in consistency so apply it several times, layer upon layer, as the previous one dries. Any of the mixture which is left over can be kept in the refrigerator and used again.

Mayonnaise Mask (for dry skin)

1 tsp mayonnaise
1 egg yolk

Nothing could be simpler than this—and it's Suzy's favourite. Beat the two ingredients together and brush on your face (with, say, a soft shaving or paint brush), rather than using your fingers. Remove as usual.

Honey Softener

1 tbsp honey
1 tbsp sour cream
1 tsp cornstarch

Mix the honey and cream together then add the cornstarch to make a thin paste. Apply with the fingertips.

Tomato Pore Cleaner

1 skinned tomato
1 tbsp powdered almonds

Mash the tomato, removing the seeds and, using only the pulp, add the powdered almonds and make a paste. Apply with your fingertips in a circular scrubbing motion. Remove with warm water and use cold milk for a final splash.

Fresh Orange and Watermelon Mask
(for normal skin)

2 slices fresh watermelon
Juice of $\frac{1}{2}$ orange
1 tbsp wholewheat flour

Remove the seeds, then mash and strain the watermelon. Mix with the orange juice and then blend the mixture with wholewheat flour. If the juice overwhelms the flour and you find the mask is very liquid, apply with cotton wool.

Papaya Peeling Mask (for all skin types)

Flesh of $\frac{1}{2}$ papaya (pawpaw)
$1\frac{1}{2}$ tsps honey

Crush the flesh of the papaya, warm the honey very slightly and mix the two together. Papaya is particularly rejuvenating and cleansing because it removes any dead cells on the skin's surface. You will find your skin literally glows after using a papaya peeling mask.

Carrot, Potato and Dried Mint Mask
(for all skin types)

1 carrot
1 potato
1 tbsp dried mint

Boil the carrot and the potato until soft and mash. Let the mix cool, then thoroughly mix in the dried mint leaves. This vegetable mask is particularly good for bringing impurities to the surface and is rich in Vitamin A.

Banana Mask (for dry skin)

1 banana
2 tbsps olive oil

Mash the banana to a paste and gradually add the oil which has first been slightly warmed. This mixture is very good for dry, parched skin as it works like a deeply-penetrating skin moisturising treatment.

Hot Oil Mask (for dry skin)

$\frac{1}{4}$ cup olive oil
$\frac{1}{4}$ cup almond oil
Piece of muslin

Cut eye, nose and mouth holes in the muslin so making a cloth mask which fits comfortably over the face. Warm the oils and dip the muslin into the hot mixture, squeeze out the excess oil and then place the muslin mask over your face. Repeat the process several times once the muslin has cooled.

Rinse off the oil with warm water and finish by wiping your face (which will still bear a fine coating of oil) with cotton wool dipped in cool milk. This treatment is excellent for aging or wind and sun dried skin.

Persimmon Mask (for any skin)

1 tbsp of flesh of ripe persimmon
A little fuller's earth

Mash the flesh of the fruit and add just enough fuller's earth to make a paste or mud-type pack. Apply as usual. The persimmon is good for any skin type as the composition of the fruit is very similar to the healthy acid quality of the skin.

Suzy's Invisible Party Mask

A film make-up artist once taught Suzy a special trick for a scene she was playing where she needed to look suddenly very young. It works for anyone who wants to look totally wrinkle-free for a special party but bear in mind that you can't move your facial muscles too much, e.g. smile, otherwise it cracks! Just take the beaten white of an egg, apply it to skin and allow it to dry. Then make up as usual on top.

Moisturisers

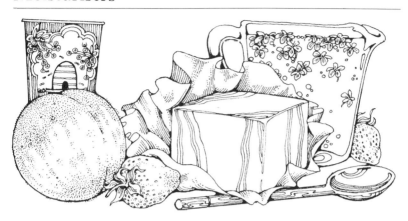

Cold weather, central heating, hot sun and piercing wind, they all rob the skin of moisture yet they are, for most of us, unavoidable facts of life. Add to these everyday problems the additional effects of the harsh, intense lights, bone-wearying, long days and endless cosmetic changes that we have both suffered while modelling and acting and it isn't hard to see why we are so deeply concerned with keeping our skins moist and young-looking and why we have tried so many different preparations.

Every skin needs moisture—and don't forget that all our recipes are just as useful to men—and one of the most basic ways of making sure both your complexion and your entire system are healthy and your eyes are bright is to drink at least eight glasses of water a day.

But your skin still needs extra help. Imagine a leaf in autumn that is so pretty that you want to dry it and keep it. If you oil the leaf before you press it, the disintegration stops and it looks once again like a fresh, new leaf. Well, your skin is the same except that it won't respond to oil alone; your complexion needs a mixture of water, oils and waxes to remain soft and well lubricated.

Oil alone, if applied to dry, chapped skin, is not effective. The skin needs water but this cannot be applied externally since it evaporates immediately. So humectants, or moisturising cream, work by creating a barrier that traps the moisture in your cells and holds it there.

One of the main problems with vegetable oils is that they consist of triglycerides which are not absorbed by the skin and, additionally, they easily go rancid. So cosmetic firms use synthetics which contain what are called unsaturated esters, which are absorbed into the skin. In our search for natural ingredients, we eventually came across a miracle plant growing in Mexico. Called Jojoba (pronounced Hohoba) it is the only vegetable oil to contain 99 per cent unsaturated esters which means it is eminently suitable for use in creams and moisturisers. As yet Jojoba is quite hard to find outside America, but it is now being grown commercially and should soon be much more readily available. We ourselves manufacture a very fine Jojoba moisturiser.

Moisturisers are much cheaper to make in your own kitchen than they are to buy in the shops and they are not overly complicated. Beeswax is an integral part of many recipes so buy it in a block, melt it all, then pour it into little teaspoon- and tablespoon-sized 'cups' made out of aluminium foil and allow to harden. This way you have the right measure of wax always available.

We believe that *how* you apply the moisturiser can be as beneficial as the cream itself, so we have included a set of simple facial massages that you can do night or morning. Do try to make them part of your routine.

1. Chin and throat:

Lightly tap the throat with the back of your hands and finger tips, working your way towards the chin. Gently slap the throat with back of hands, keeping a rhythmic movement.

2. Double chins:

With the thumb and first finger of each hand quickly pinch above the jawbone working from the hairline towards the chin, then repeat under the jaw on softer flesh. Good for firming the entire soft chin area.

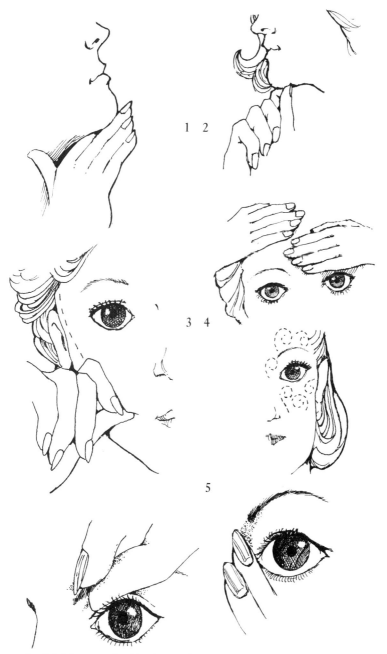

Facial Massages for Putting on Moisturiser

3. Firming the face:

Repeat the above pinching movement starting at the mouth and working up the cheekbones to the hairline. Good for circulation.

4. Forehead wrinkles and lines:

With flat hands make a firm stroking motion from the top of nose towards the hairline over the forehead, one hand after the other, rhythmically repeating for several moments.

5. Eye area:

To increase circulation and keep skin looking alive, pinch along both eyebrows with your thumb and first finger in quick movements. For tension and headaches, with your middle two fingers press in the hollow of corner of eyes, then move on at half inch spots, putting pressure on for a moment and then releasing.

When either making up or putting on nightcream or moisturiser, always use circular movements beginning at the nose, following over the browbone then circling under the eyes, back towards the nose. This is contrary to the way most people apply creams to the eye area but is the correct method to avoid wrinkling.

Ideally, these movements should be done every day but at least make sure that the general upwards and circling movements become a habit when applying makeup or creams.

One of the glaring mistakes many people make in good faith is to cover their faces and neck in thick creams at night in the belief the cream will 'sink in' while they sleep. Unfortunately, this is a passport to wrinkles because the facial muscles don't work much at night. The skin can only absorb so much and that limit occurs about ten to twenty minutes after applying the cream. So before you go to sleep remember to blot thoroughly your face and neck with a clean tissue, removing any surplus. This is particularly important for the delicate eye area. A skin specialist told us that any oil or grease left under the eyes at night creates bags and wrinkles as the downward pull of the heavy grease makes folds and lines, which is not exactly the desired effect for any of us. So always gently reblot the area under the eyes.

A good tip for those with particularly dry skin is to keep handy a spray filled with mild rosewater and lightly spray your face after applying any moisturiser or cream. This not only momentarily hydrates the skin but also helps the cream to penetrate.

Avocado Basic Moisturiser

2 tsps beeswax
1 tsp emulsifying wax
2 tsps almond oil
3 tsps avocado oil
4 tbsps rosewater

Melt the waxes in a bowl placed in a larger pan of water so that the heat is indirect and the melting process is slow. When ready add the two oils to the melted waxes. In another bowl heat the rosewater in the same pan of hot water so that the contents of both bowls are at the same temperature. Slowly, drop by drop, add the rosewater to the oil and wax mixture, constantly stirring with a wooden spoon. Remove the now complete mixture from the heat and keep stirring until it sets.

Simple Peach Moisturiser

3 tbsps lanolin
3 tbsps almond oil
3 tbsps peach juice

Melt the lanolin and the oil together and then add the juice from fresh peaches. Remove from the heat and stir very hard. Instead of fresh peach juice, you can substitute strawberry juice or cucumber juice.

Violet Moisturising Cream

1 oz olive oil
1 tbsp anhydrous lanolin
1 egg yolk
¼ tsp violet extract (take a handful of violet flowers, and
   pour over them two ozs of boiling water. Leave for
   two hours, then strain)
½ tsp liquid lecithin

Melt the lanolin over a low heat. In a separate pan
warm the oil and lecithin, remove from the heat, then slowly
beat the mixture into the warmed lanolin until it looks
creamy and has cooled. Beat the egg yolk and violet extract
into the cream and keep beating until it is fluffy. Refrigerate
immediately.

Honey and Orange Moisturising Lotion

3 tbsps anhydrous lanolin
2 tbsps cocoa butter
1 tsp coconut oil
1 tbsp safflower oil
1 tsp honey
1 oz orange oil
½ tsp liquid lecithin

Melt the lanolin and cocoa butter slowly, then add the
honey. In a separate saucepan warm the coconut oil, lecithin
and safflower oil together and, pouring a drop at a time, beat
this into the other mixture. Finally add the orange oil,
beating all the time until the consistency is creamy. Allow to
cool, put in a jar or empty cosmetic tub and refrigerate.

Cucumber Moisturiser

1 tbsp beeswax
2 ozs safflower oil
½ tsp liquid lecithin
2 tbsps cucumber juice

1 tbsp rosewater
$\frac{1}{8}$ tsp borax

Wash a quarter of a cucumber and blend the whole thing, skin and all, until you have 2 tbsps juice. Heat it but do not allow it to boil and set aside. Melt the beeswax over a low heat, separately warm the safflower oil and lecithin and beat these two ingredients into the heated wax. Slowly reheat the cucumber juice with the rosewater and borax and slowly beat this into the wax and oil mixture until cool and creamy. Keep in the fridge.

Elderflower Moisturiser

2 tbsps emulsifying wax
1 tbsp almond oil
1 tbsp sunflower oil
1 tsp lanolin
$\frac{1}{2}$ tsp borax
1 tsp witch hazel
$1\frac{1}{4}$ tsps glycerine
8 tbsps elderflower water

Take a handful of elderflower blossoms and steep in a covered pot, in just the same way you would make tea. Set aside to cool, then strain. Melt the waxes together in a small pan or pudding basin set inside a larger one containing simmering water. In a separate bowl heat the borax, glycerine, strained elderflower water and witch hazel. Take off the heat and add the liquid to the oils, stirring very thoroughly all the time until cool. The result should be a non-greasy skin cream with a refreshing scent.

Anti-Wrinkle Treatments and Eye Care

One of our first experiments with making anti-wrinkle cream was when Vitamin E became available in capsules. We began to break them into the nightcream we were currently using.

Vitamin E put directly on the eye area is too heavy for the delicate skin but when contained in a cream it helps ease wrinkle lines.

A dermatologist told us of a simple exercise for eyes which is very beneficial and helps keep the muscle tone. Just screw up your eyes very tightly then open them as widely as possible and focus far away. Repeat 100 times.

Most people either ignore or abuse their best asset—their eyes. They are not prepared to treat these 'windows of the soul' with the gentleness and care they deserve and they groan every time a wrinkle appears. The reason that the very fine skin around the eye area does wrinkle faster than the rest of the face is that there are no oil glands around the eyes, so it is essential that the skin is kept moist, then the lines and crinkles won't deepen as quickly. Try to use as little powder as possible around your eyes.

Take the trouble to use a suitable cream around your eyes at night, and remember what we said earlier—all night creams should be well-blotted before you go to sleep.

When applying makeup, never try to cover over wrinkles and lines—it won't work, instead it will emphasise your age as the makeup cakes in the lines. Use a generous amount of moisturiser on wrinkles and very little makeup base and, if possible, no powder. Try it on your own face—use a lot of makeup around one eye and thin it to practically nothing around the other. Powder the one eye, then after half an hour take another look. The moist skin around the eye will still be young-looking, while the other area will not be as attractive. In principle, the older you are the less makeup you should use.

Simple Strawberry Rejuvenating Cream

2 tbsps butter that has been kept in warm room
1 tbsp strawberry juice (made from pressing fresh
    strawberries through sieve after being washed)

Mix the juice of the fruit with the softened butter until

you have a creamy consistency. Use immediately, putting the 'cream' on your face and neck for ten minutes and then wash it off with warm water, followed by a cold splash. This 'cream' should not be left on overnight, you might end up smelling rancid!

Easy Night Cream

2 tbsps white petroleum jelly
4 tbsps anhydrous lanolin
2 tbsps almond oil

Warm the lanolin and the petroleum jelly in a pudding basin placed in a pan of hot water and mix well. Remove from heat. Beat firmly until cool, add the oil and keep beating vigorously until the consistency seems creamy. Keep in a screwtop jar.

Vitamin Cream for Dry Skin

6 tbsps Easy Night Cream (recipe above)
3 capsules Vitamin A or E

Prick the capsules with a needle and mix well into your homemade cream until all the vitamin oil has disappeared into the cream. This bonus for dry skin is best absorbed when taking a long bath. Afterwards wipe off the cream and splash your face and neck with a tonic.

Wrinkle Softener

$1\frac{1}{2}$ tbsps anhydrous lanolin
$2\frac{1}{2}$ tsps coconut oil
4 tbsps wheatgerm oil

Melt the lanolin and coconut oil together. Heat the wheatgerm oil separately and when warm beat into the lanolin mixture. Keep beating constantly until the cream thickens.

Warm Olive Oil Treatment

For dark shadows or pouches under the eyes, dip some cotton wool in warm olive oil and stroke gently under your eyes. Leave on and rest for fifteen minutes, remove the oil gently with warm water, then splash with a toner. You can also do this when you are applying a mask.

Honey Anti-Wrinkle Lotion

1 tbsp glycerine
1 tbsp rosewater
1 tbsp witch hazel
2 tbsps clear honey

No cooking is involved with this recipe, you just thoroughly mix together all the ingredients and store in a bottle or jar. It's a very pleasant and effective recipe to counter wrinkled skin but it can be a little sticky, so we suggest you use it on your face and neck during the daytime when you're alone and you can tie your hair off your face.

Fennel Instant Wrinkle Relief

Simply soak fennel leaves in rosewater for one hour. Lie down and lay the soaked leaves across your face for fifteen minutes—try and doze, resting never hurt wrinkles.

Clear Eye Tips

Sleep, in fact, is one of the most important keys to a glowing complexion and bright eyes. But many people find sleep evades them as they turn over the worries of the day, real or imagined. Suzy used to qualify as a bona fide insomniac and she counted more sheep than most people have had hot dinners. But to no avail. Then she discovered what works for her—she thinks of a happy day in her life and recounts it to herself in immense detail, remembering, say, even the scent of the flowers in the room. Now she has beaten her sleeping problem and she never gets to midday in her remembrances because she has always dropped off by then. The trick is total concentration—then your mind can't 'wander' back to problems.

Diet is also very important for the eyes as well as the skin and the more fresh vegetables you can eat, the better. Puffiness around the eyes can be the result of a bad diet, or too little sleep or as we said earlier, the result of too much cream left on the eye area, or even a dry atmosphere. For instance, if you have central heating but no humidifier, try putting a bowl of water in front of your radiators.

We both swear by pads of cotton wool soaked in cucumber toner on our eyes while we try to relax but other people just put slices of fresh cucumber straight on their eyelids. Used teabags are a favourite of some, once again applied directly to closed eyes while resting. Pat's grandmother used always to keep an infusion of a herb called eyebright in a cold place and claimed it had wondrous properties for dark circles and tired eyes. A camomile infusion is another age-old eye aid which is very soothing.

For inflamed, red eyes cook two cored, peeled apples in a little water and when cool put the mixture in squares of muslin and place on your eyes while you rest.

Try all or any of these ideas but don't forget, you mustn't lie there and worry while the cucumber or the camomile is working otherwise you'll defeat the purpose. Relaxation is all important.

Always be extra gentle when touching the eye area, never pull or stretch the skin and try taking off your eye makeup with castor oil. Then when you have gently tissued off the makeup, reapply a little castor oil to your lashes with an old, clean mascara brush. Regular use makes lashes very lustrous and thick.

Skin Problems

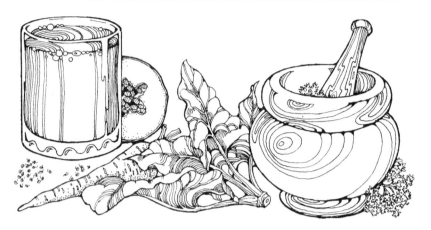

Diet, nervousness, lack of sleep and improper cleansing can all create spots, blackheads and nasty bumps. Acne is usually the result of a hormonal imbalance.

We all know what we should eat and what we should avoid but it doesn't stop us tucking into chips and chocolate from time to time. So if you are prone to any skin imperfections, clean up your act—literally, in the care you take with daily cleansing routines, and figuratively, in the care you take with the food you put into your body. Exercise and fresh air will also help.

Apart from eating lots of fresh vegetables and salads, drink straight vegetable juices, carrot, spinach or lettuce, or mix any or all of them into a vegetable cocktail. And don't forget to drink plenty of water. A drink of warm water and fresh lemon juice, first thing in the morning, is a great cleanser.

If you are eating right but are inclined to be constipated, that condition can contribute to blemishes. So take a mild laxative to rid yourself of toxins and impurities or, even better, begin a morning breakfast ritual which should keep you regular. Six prunes, two large spoons of bran and a banana cut up in a bowl of milk is nutritious, full of fibre and Vitamin A.

Parsley when eaten is a mild diuretic. For spots press the juice out of the parsley and apply it directly to the infected area. It also works on insect bites and stings.

Be very careful if you decide to clean out a blackhead or squeeze a spot. Always steam your face first and take a fresh tissue in each hand to remove the blemish. If light pressure doesn't remove it, leave it for another time. Pressure of this sort can damage the under layers of the skin. Once you have removed the offensive object, dab the area with antiseptic or tonic. And don't pick. There's nothing worse for your skin than absent-minded probing.

Avoid makeup if your skin is erupting, it is bound to make it worse, and stay away from coffee and alcohol, they just aggravate the condition. And remember what we said earlier—don't use a harsh astringent.

Blackhead Scrub

Handful of alfalfa sprouts
1 oz oatmeal

Pound the alfalfa sprouts or put them in a blender, and mix with the oatmeal to make a paste. Apply this to your face and leave on for 15 minutes. Rinse off with milk then splash with cold water.

Yoghurt Cleanser

Apply a mask of natural yoghurt daily, leave on for ten minutes, and then rinse off.

Pawpaw Cleanser

Mash the pawpaw to a pulp, apply once a week for ten minutes and rinse off.

(Both the above cleansers 'eat away' the impurities of the skin.)

Antiseptic Mask

If you have gently squeezed out blackheads, apply a paste of kaolin and a few drops of ten volume peroxide for five minutes. Do not leave this mask on any longer as the properties are very harsh.

If after eating right, keeping your skin scrupulously clean and taking plenty of walks in the fresh air your skin is still bad, see your doctor or dermatologist.

Hands and Feet

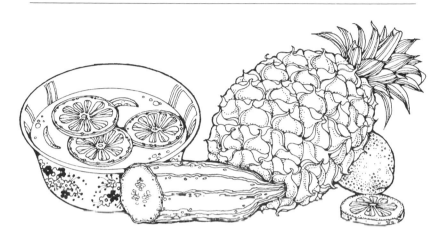

It used to be said that you could tell a lady by her hands, which meant of course that ladies did not work and so had soft, smooth hands. Well, these days women frequently both do the housework and have a job, so our hands could do with a little help.

Lemon is a natural for hands (and elbows) because it acts as a slight bleach and combined with any oil makes a perfect protection against detergents and harsh treatment which roughens the skin. This citrus fruit is also a vital ingredient in a simple but effective hand softening lotion.

Lemon Hand Milk

1 slice of lemon
$\frac{1}{2}$ cup milk

Let the slice of lemon sit in the milk for about three hours or until the milk has begun to curdle. Remove the lemon and use the milk regularly as a skin feeding and softening lotion. Refrigerate when not being used.

Glycerine and Rosewater Hand Lotion

4 ozs rosewater
4 ozs glycerine
$\frac{3}{4}$ oz borax

Dissolve the borax in warmed rosewater and beat into the warmed glycerine until cool. Bottle the mixture and shake before using.

Cucumber Hand Lotion

3″ piece of peeled cucumber, chopped and mashed
1 tbsp witch hazel
1 tsp glycerine
1 tsp rosewater

Put the ingredients in a blender for 30 seconds, bottle and keep in the fridge. This lotion is particularly nice when used icy cold. If you're feeling extravagant, it also makes a wonderful body lotion in warm weather.

Peach Hand Cream

2 ozs almond oil
2 ozs peach kernel oil
$1\frac{1}{2}$ tsps beeswax

Mix the two oils. In a small saucepan over a low heat melt the wax to which a little of the oil mixture has been added. Keep taking the pan off the heat so the wax doesn't burn. As soon as it is nearly softened add the rest of the oil mixture, constantly stirring with a wooden spoon. Remove from the heat and keep stirring until cool. This peach cream is extra rich and protects the hands very well from the rigours of housework.

Pineapple Nail Soak

To strengthen the nails and soften the skin around

them, simply soak your finger tips in a bowl of pineapple juice. You can re-use the juice for a second nail soak if you keep it in the fridge but allow it to return to room temperature before you put your fingers in it.

Feet are frequently one of the most neglected parts of the body. Some of us may bother to polish our toenails in the summer but very few of us actually take care of our feet, which is a little short-sighted when you consider how much we rely on them. You should change shoe heights during the day several times as this exercises different muscles with each pair of shoes, and always try to go barefoot for at least part of the day. When moving around the house, make a point of sometimes walking on tiptoe, as this helps circulation and is good for the bones in the feet. When watching television or reading, curl and uncurl the toes, it will keep your feet supple and strong. You can use your hand lotion on your feet, too, to soften them.

If your feet are sunburned or tired, soak a sliced cucumber in milk for one hour, then place it on your feet. The cucumber is slightly astringent and the milk is soothing.

If your feet are particularly tired, try soaking them for 20 minutes in lukewarm water into which $\frac{1}{2}$ a lemon has been sliced. Rub your soles and heels (and any callouses) with the lemon slices, rinse and powder. Then rest your feet on a pillow or cushion, so that they are slightly higher than the rest of the body.

Sun and Skin

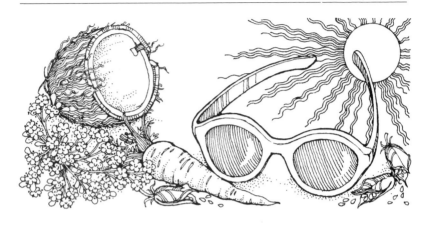

We all know by now that over-exposure to the sun is bad for the skin but most of us still don't know when we've had enough. Sunburn is very sneaky, you never feel it until it's too late. Before you go out in the sun take Vitamin B tablets, especially those containing PABA, if you can get it, which are supposed to protect the skin from harmful rays. One friend swears by taking a course of Vitamin A capsules before she plans to get a tan; she says it takes the pain out of the process. Another way of doing this would be to eat a lot of carrots, which have a high Vitamin A content.

When you sunbathe, do keep your skin soft by using a lotion or oil, and of course take it gently at first.

Sensitive Skin Tanning Oil

2 parts coconut oil
1 part sesame oil
Few drops of sandalwood oil

Warm the coconut oil and the sesame oil together, remove from heat and add a few drops of sandalwood oil. Beat all the ingredients together and keep beating so they don't separate. Shake well before use.

Tanning Oil for Normal Skin

Equal parts of cocoa butter and coconut oil
Few drops of sandalwood oil

Make as above, beat well.

Sun Oil for Tanned Skin

Even when you have a tan, your skin still needs lubrication.
We've found that a mixture of two parts of olive oil and
one part of vinegar mixed and shaken well is the best skin
softener. Ignore anyone who says you smell like a salad!

If after this you still overdo it and end up with a slight
case of sunburn, try our

Elderflower Soother

3 handfuls of fresh elderflower blossoms
4 ozs lard

Put the lard and the blossoms together over a low heat
and warm gently, stirring constantly, for 20 minutes. Strain
through a sieve and keep in a screwtop jar until needed. If
you have the kind of skin that burns then make this recipe in
advance of sunbathing and keep it ready for when you need it.

Prickly Heat Relief

Try a tablespoon of bicarbonate of soda in your bathwater
and if you go back out into the sun, mix vinegar into your
sun lotion or even just apply vinegar directly to the skin. It's
very soothing and the smell does evaporate quite quickly.

Sunburn Coolers

If just your face is burned, halve two strawberries and rub
them over your face. Leave on the residue of the juice for 30
minutes then wash off with warm water into which has been
added a few drops of tincture of benzoin.

As Suzy found when she was filming, if you go a nasty
shade of red or pink in the face through over-exposure, the
best thing to do is to rub a little yoghurt into your skin and
let it dry. Make sure you wash it off thoroughly with
lukewarm water. Yoghurt is very good for toning down
redness.

A nice, simple skin lotion for sunburn can be made by
packing elderflower blossoms into an earthenware jar,
covering them with boiling water and letting them cool.
Then add 3 tbsps alcohol. Cover the jar with a cloth and
leave in a warm place for six hours, then strain and bottle.

Mouth and Teeth

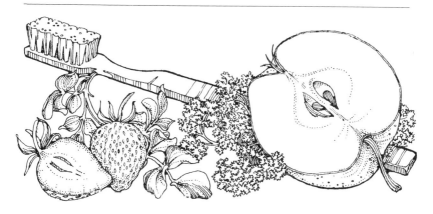

A natural way of cleaning the breath is to eat parsley—it also has the added advantage of being cleansing to the whole digestive system. For soft or bleeding gums, chew watercress, which also has the beneficial effect of helping make the skin clear.

To make a freshening mouthwash, take several sprigs of watercress, soak them in half a pint of boiling water, cool, strain and use cold from refrigerator.

A healing mouthwash can be made by simmering the seeds of quince in boiling water, strain and cool then use.

If you want another breath freshener that doesn't even need boiling, take one cup of apple juice (unsweetened) and swirl it around your mouth for a couple of minutes. You can, of course, simply put a cored apple in the blender and make your own juice.

To keep your teeth white, try rubbing the juice of fresh strawberries on your teeth and leaving it on for three minutes. It helps remove stains and discolorations. Afterwards, rinse your mouth with warm water in which you have mixed a pinch of bicarbonate of soda.

Baths

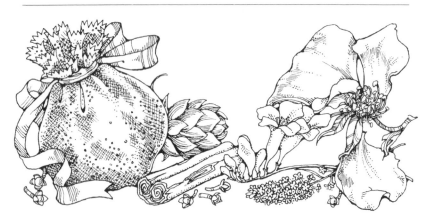

Taking a bath should be a pleasing experience but too many people don't allow the time and don't bother to make the bathroom an attractive place in which to lounge around. Suzy's bathroom has two light switches, one that operates a central bright light and another that turns on two antique lamps which send out a soft, rosy glow. So she can lie in a bath filled with the scent of herbs in a low light or turn on the intensity of a bright bulb when she wants to clean her face thoroughly or apply makeup.

Suzy is something of a bath nut, it's where she retreats to solve her problems. Once, when she had trekked for six days across the plains of Peru encountering only the most primitive sanitation, she suddenly saw a large, modern American-style hotel looming on the horizon. She headed straight for the bathroom where she spent two hours and that hotel has remained fondly in her memories ever since.

Pat has papered her bathroom with rich, dark colours, hung plants in pretty pots, it's where she stores many of her herbs in heavy, earthenware jars, and she leaves sprigs, tied with ribbon, hanging round her mirror to give the room a permanently delightful scent. When Pat first started picking the herbs that were growing in country hedgerows, she used to throw them in the bath whole, which works perfectly well.

As she became more knowledgeable, however, she realised she was wasting these lovely blossoms and leaves, so now she makes up little muslin sachets, containing a mixture of several different herbs, that hang from her taps and automatically scent the water as the bath fills. All you need do is to combine any of the following list of herbs, picking them for the aromas that please you most: lavender, basil, mint, lemon balm, thyme, marjoram, comfrey, rosemary and yarrow.

Suzy keeps jars by the bath so that she has anything she might need to hand. Oatmeal, for instance, for getting rid of dead cells (rub handfuls of it on your skin), dried milk for a milk bath, vinegar for when her skin feels irritated, honey for relieving tiredness, rosewater which goes in her baby daughter's bath, and a large jar of mixed, healing herbs.

Pat has found that a wonderful aid for dry skin is to mash up cinnamon sticks and warm them in baby oil with a dozen cloves, and leave for several days. She then removes the cloves and puts the oil and cinnamon sticks into a pretty bottle and uses a little whenever she finds she needs it. Plain eucalyptus oil in the bath is very effective against dry skin as well.

If her skin gets rough in winter Pat packs oatmeal into sachets with a few herbs and after running the water over the sachets, she rubs them over her body, using the sachets like a gentle, sweet-smelling loofah.

Both of us believe in hunting through junk shops for pretty, old bottles and jars which you can still find for a few pence. Wash them out and keep them on display full of the ingredients you need—they are also a cheap and attractive way of decorating a rather plain bathroom or kitchen.

Milk baths have been around since Cleopatra who, as we all know, was very partial to asses' milk. Since asses are scarce today and milk on this scale is expensive, try putting a handful of powdered milk into your bath water. It does work and you will feel more pampered than you might imagine.

Lemon-Almond Bath Oil

2 ozs lemon extract
4 ozs almond oil
2 drops yellow food colouring*

Put ingredients into a pretty bottle and shake well.
Shake before each use. Refrigerate.

(*Food colouring is not a 'must' in these recipes for bath oil, but
it does make the mixture look very attractive.)

Garden Fresh Bath Oil

1 handful rose petals (or any other flower that smells
    good from your garden)
2 ozs glycerine (has no smell)
2 drops pink food colouring

Leave the flower petals to stand in the glycerine for
about a week. Strain off the petals, add the other ingredients
and shake well. Pour this delightful smelling oil into a pretty,
old bottle.

This basic method can be adopted to any flowers of
your choice, we have found freesias and lavender are
particularly suitable substitutes for roses. If you can't be
bothered with letting the petals sit in the glycerine for a
week, then simply add a few drops of your favourite
perfume. The advantage of this method is that the scent of
the bath oil will not conflict with any perfume you usually
spray on when dressed. After your bath, rub your body with
a little of the bath oil instead of using a body lotion.

Herbal Healing Baths

Herbal baths are very relaxing, so try to take one before you
go to bed or rest. Take a herb or a mixture of several herbs,
steep for several hours in two pints of water just as you
would if making a strong cup of tea, strain and then add the
entire two pints to your bath. The healing herbs we

recommend are parsley, sage, basil, mint and yarrow.

For anyone who has trouble sleeping, a herbal healing bath does wonders. Pat makes herbal sleep pillows from hops, mixed with lavender and rosemary. She fills a 12″ square pillow with this mixture and leaves it among her bed pillows all the time. The hops are very soporific. If you just want a sweet-smelling pillow, leave out the hops and substitute lemon balm or thyme.

Hair

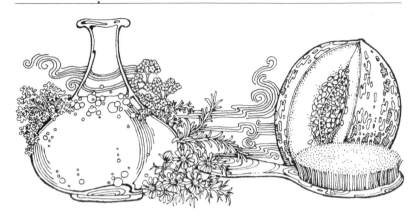

We have all been brought up to believe that our hair should be our crowning glory, which probably accounts for so many people being so chronically depressed over what they see in the mirror. Few of us have thick, bouncy hair of bright blonde or perfect raven colour but we can all make the most of what we do have. All it takes is understanding.

The hair is made up of several layers, covered by a protective outer layer known as the epicuticle. Unfortunately this outer layer is itself easily damaged and when you see hair that has a fuzzy look to its surface, then the epicuticle has not been treated right.

Some types of hair are much more vulnerable than others and, needless to say, that thick, bouncy kind that we all envy is also the most resilient. But understanding your own hair type and its limitations is a good start to better-looking hair.

Since both of us have had our hair dyed every colour of the rainbow, endured perms and bleaching and tight wigs, we are very aware that as natural blondes we have fine hair that needs nourishing. Few people have hair that can for years take the trauma of bleaching and colouring, and, fundamentally, most hair is best only taken a shade or so lighter or darker than its natural colour.

Try not to overdo the use of electric rollers or hair

dryers, they are both very drying. Whenever possible let your hair dry naturally in the sun, for your scalp produces Vitamin D which is very healthy.

The old adage about 100 strokes a day does, actually, hold good. Our grandmothers were right. Bend forward from the waist and brush from the roots to the ends thus distributing evenly the sheen from the oils at the roots. Follow every stroke with your hand to eliminate electricity. Only if you have an oily scalp is brushing a bad idea, it just over-activates your already over-active oil glands.

Basically, your hair is a barometer of your general health and depression; tiredness or illness can alter its appearance. But what you eat is very important—as we've already said—and a diet that is comprised of lean meat, salads and fresh vegetables will do your hair as much good as it will benefit your figure. Potatoes, carrots, watercress and the white part of leeks are all particularly good for healthy hair. Junk food just makes for drab, lifeless hair.

Taking brewers' yeast tablets every day gives a shine to your hair—after all that's what show dogs are fed to get their coats in tip-top condition! Six or seven tablets a day is what most hairdressers agree to be the necessary amount.

We believe that hair, like skin, should be treated gently and that mild shampoos and natural treatments and rinses used as often as *your* hair type needs them are best.

For years Pat was fanatical about trying to straighten her wavy hair, in the days when those perfect, straight bobs were in style. Now she has confronted the fact that her hair is fine, naturally wavy and inclined to be unmanageable, so instead of unsuccessfully trying to tame it she has learned to make the most of it. She has it layered to give it volume and lets it follow its own inclinations and wave where it will. When she's working in hot lights she leaves a little conditioner, or even puts a few drops of baby oil, on the ends to stop breakage. To give it plenty of body she never combs or brushes it through completely until it is dry. Instead she pinches and pats it in an upward movement, pushing it into shape with her fingers.

So instead of sighing over magazine pictures of other people's hair (after all, we *know* that many of those styles would only hold up on us for a matter of an hour), accept the limitations of your own hair type and set about making it as healthy and pretty a frame for your face as possible.

Making your own shampoo is quite difficult, as we've discovered through trial and error, and we suggest that you first buy a mild shampoo (baby shampoo is good) and dilute it further with herbal infusions—yarrow for greasy hair, rosemary if you have dandruff, camomile for fair hair, sage for brunettes and parsley or thyme for any type.

You can also enrich a very mild shop-bought shampoo by whisking an egg into it. Then you have instant protein and instant enrichment. If your hair is very dry or damaged, then shampoo with eggs alone. Beat two or three eggs together until fluffy and work them into wet hair, wait about ten minutes before rinsing. Be sure that the water is not hot, otherwise you will end up with unappetising scrambled egg all over your head.

If you suddenly have to go out when your hair needs washing, don't panic. Suzy was once saved by a hairdresser on a film set when she was suddenly invited to a producer's party. She had been wearing a flattening, hot wig all day. The hairdresser simply parted her own, lank hair into small sections and rubbed a little baby powder into the hairline, then brushed it out thoroughly. The result, she says, was very good, although she would only recommend you do this in a crisis.

After shampooing and rinsing your hair, it's time to add a beneficial final rinse made from herbs. For these we suggest you make strong infusions, just as you would with a strong pot of tea, and use two bowls so that you can catch the infusion in the second bowl and pour it back over your hair several times.

For greasy hair use Peruvian bark, yarrow, verbena, marigold or sage; for fair hair, which is usually drier, use camomile, lemon balm or lavender; comfrey is suitable for any hair type; and those with dandruff should try nettles or rosemary as well as comfrey. Melon also works well on oily hair. Mash and blend ¼ melon (without skin) and allow the juice to stay on your hair for five minutes. Then rinse out. Beer makes a good final rinse if you want your hair to have more body. Just dilute it with equal parts of water. And if you've had a special party and anyone has left a glass of champagne sitting around until it's gone flat, then that's a wonderful final rinse. Though we'd be tempted to drink it instead!

Vinegar Final Rinse

Dilute the vinegar—about eight parts water to one part vinegar—and keep a bottle ready in the bathroom. Vinegar adds gloss and lights, particularly to dark hair.

Lemon Rinse

Blondes should dilute lemon juice in the same proportions as above and it works in the same way as vinegar, leaving hair very shiny. If you are in the sun and you want to lighten your fair hair, towel dry, then pour on four parts of water to one part fresh lemon juice. Dry your hair in the sun and you will see the highlights come up. Never use straight, undiluted lemon juice as a bleach, it's sticky and very harsh on the hair.

Sage Rinse

To intensify the colour of dark hair and bring out highlights, steep a handful of sage leaves in 1 qt boiling water for two hours, then strain. Pour over your hair repeatedly and leave on for twenty minutes. Then wash out with clear water.

Conditioning treatments are very important and should be used regularly. Honey is probably the most basic and effective but it's also rather sticky and hard to remove. So we suggest you use oil instead and that you steam your hair so that it really penetrates. Once again, throw some herbs (lemon balm or mint) in the steam water and clean your face at the same time. But don't forget to close your pores afterward, before you do anything else to your hair.

Hot Oil Treatment

2–3 ozs warm olive oil (for dry hair) or 2–3 ozs
   almond oil (for greasy hair)

Shampoo your hair, then towel lightly. Section your hair and distribute the oil from the roots to the ends, paying special attention to the ends which usually need it most. Massage well. Then steam your hair with a towel over your head and a bowl of hot water and herbs for ten minutes. Shampoo your hair again and rinse.

High Protein Treatment

2 eggs
1 tbsp lemon juice or vinegar

Beat the eggs with the lemon juice or vinegar until fluffy. Work into wet, clean hair and leave on for 15 minutes. Rinse out thoroughly with lukewarm water and make a final rinse of your choice.

Dandruff Treatment

1 tsp borax
1 cup warm rosewater

Mix the ingredients together. Brush your hair, then wet the brush with the solution and brush your scalp with it. Repeat.

Hair Tonic

Handful of artichoke leaves

Simmer the leaves for several hours in a covered pot, cool and when ready to use the tonic strain it and rub it into scalp. Any leftovers can be stored in the fridge.

Tonic for Thinning Hair

Make a very strong infusion of Peruvian bark, allow it to cool and pour over your head using the two-basin method so that it goes through the hair several times. Peruvian bark promotes hair growth.

Tonic for Dull Hair

2 egg yolks
2 tsps gin

Beat the yolks into the gin until it all froths. Massage well into the scalp and rinse thoroughly with warm water. You won't need to shampoo as the egg yolk cleans hair as well as making it shine.

Tonic for Dull and Dandruffy Hair

$\frac{1}{2}$ cup white wine vinegar
$\frac{1}{2}$ cup water

Shake together in a bottle, then gently massage into the scalp with flannels or cloths soaked in the solution. Repeat two or three times a week before shampooing.

Treatment for Excessively Dry Hair

$\frac{1}{3}$ ripe avocado
$\frac{1}{3}$ cup mayonnaise

This treatment Suzy got from her sister, Mary. Mix the two ingredients together until really smooth. Massage the mixture into the scalp, cover your head with a shower cap and leave for $\frac{1}{2}$—1 hour. Rinse out well, shampoo normally.

Remember that wet hair is very breakable and should only be approached with caution. Use a wide-toothed comb and work from the ends if there are any tangles to deal with. Never pull, take a small section and gradually work your way up to the roots.

If you have a style that needs setting, sugar is one of the simplest natural setting lotions. Take one heaped tablespoon of sugar to one cup of boiling water and when the sugar has dissolved and the mixture cooled, use to set hair. One teaspoon of plain gelatin to one cup of boiling water has the same effect.

If you like to use a lacquer, put one of these sets in a bottle with a fine spray top and use sparingly.

8 Questions

In the course of setting up our business, and experimenting with various recipes, we have often been asked for advice and ideas on a wide variety of topics. As many people often have the same sort of questions, here are twenty of them, with our answers, which deal with miscellaneous items we couldn't touch on in the text itself.

Q. Why have I been told by so many magazine articles to take Vitamin C regularly?

A. This vitamin cannot be stored in the body so it's vital to have a daily intake. Amongst its other benefits, Vitamin C is a natural diuretic. It's found in citrus fruits and if you can bear to eat the pith, that is the most nutritious part of the fruit. Also found in strawberries and tomatoes.

Q. I have recently found liver spots on my hands, is there anything I can do about them?

A. Experts have told us that a good Vitamin B complex supplement will help but you also have to remember to maintain a balanced diet. We don't recommend bleaching creams as they can cause long-term irritation of the skin. Some pointers: it's a help not to go out in the sun without maximum protection, and never use a sun tan preparation that contains bergamot. And *never* go out in the sun having applied perfume to exposed areas, as this can really discolour your skin.

Q. Even though I use rollers, I still can't give body to my fine hair.

A. We know of a model girl who swears by this method: she waits till her hair is nearly dry then twists each section into a long coil before placing on the roller.

Q. I've been reading your brochure and I see you don't have a hormone cream. Why?

A. We feel dealing with hormones is a tricky business best left to a doctor and as all preparations put on your body do enter the system, and as certain hormones have side effects such as superfluous hair, we don't want our clients to end up with wonderful skin but also horrible hairy patches.

Q. Pat, I read in a magazine that you do yoga to keep you fit. It all seems rather complicated, can you suggest which exercises make a good basic routine?

A. Yoga is very simple, although some positions are difficult to achieve. The whole idea of it is to make you feel more serene, calm and in control and I do find a daily workout of 20 minutes or so has that effect. I would suggest you start with a general stretching exercise, feet about 3 ft apart, then gently allow your body to fall forward and bounce up and down with arms straight in front of you. Sway first over one foot, then over the other, trying to get your hands flat on the floor. This will loosen up your legs, your torso and your arms and will improve your circulation. Remember that yoga should be a series of fluid, gentle movements, so never strain yourself.
Next I would pick the Lotus position, which loosens the legs and feet, reduces flabbiness on thighs and bottom and creates a harmonious, relaxed feeling in the entire body. Sit on the floor with your legs out in front of you, place your right foot so that it rests on the upper part of your left thigh, then place your left foot against the right thigh, so that it is in the fold of the right leg. Straighten your back, put your hands on your knees, hold this

position for several minutes and try to relax, breathing deeply.

As a last basic exercise, try the Cobra. Lie on your stomach on the floor, rest your forehead on floor and place your fingers under your shoulders, hands facing each other. Very, very slowly tilt the head backwards and raise the torso by pushing down on your hands. Then slowly arch the spine and continue the movement backwards until your torso is upright, your head and shoulders leaning back and your thighs and legs are still flat on the floor. Slowly lower yourself back to the floor, keeping your spine arched, arms at sides, relax and repeat.

This movement firms the upper body, strengthens arms and buttocks and helps remove tension from the back and the neck.

If, after a few days of trying these exercises, you enjoy yoga, then it would be worth buying a book on the subject as each position needs explanation of its subtleties and benefits.

Q. My nails have been splitting horizontally, can you suggest what I am doing wrong?

A. You are filing them too low down at the sides of your nails. Try and let them grow in a more square shape, and you could also try our hints on pineapple juice or almond oil as a soak.

Q. Is there any natural deodorant that I can make myself?

A. Make an infusion with a handful of lavender in a half a pint of boiling water, steep for a day, strain. Use under arms (and it smells delicious).

Q. There are so many different diets that talk about low cholesterol, what are the basics I should know to keep down my own cholesterol level?

A. Use margarines instead of butter, eat lots of fresh vegetables and salads, if you must eat meat grill it and cut off the fat but have it no more than once a day. It's far better to substitute fish a few times a week. Don't eat cheese or eggs too often and try to stick to skimmed milk.

Q. I don't use suntan lotion very often and I'm worried about the shelf life of the one I bought. How long does it last?

A. The average life is three years but if you just mix oil and vinegar together it's a very simple and effective way of making your own. Just shake these ingredients together.

Q. Can you tell me if you have found a natural breath freshener?

A. Yes, eat an apple and it cleans your teeth, too.

Q. Is there anything I can do to make my eyelashes grow longer?

A. Try castor oil, applied at night after cleansing with a clean mascara brush.

Q. I have a very fair skin and, however careful I am, I always seem to feel uncomfortable after my first day in the sun, even when I'm not actually burned.

A. Try taking a tepid bath afterwards, you should find it very soothing to your skin.

Q. What do you consider to be the most important vitamins and what do you find them in?

A. All vitamins are useful but we'd pick Vitamin A which is found in high proportions in fresh liver, butter and oils, milk, egg yolk, fish and watercress; Vitamin B

complex, which comes in Brewer's yeast, liver,
wheatgerm, cereals, beans and lentils; Vitamin C which
comes in oranges, lemons, strawberries, tomatoes and
green peppers; Vitamin D which you find in eggs, butter,
codliver oil and from sunbathing; and Vitamin E
which is contained in wheatgerm, leafy vegetables, and
unprocessed vegetable oils and cereals.

Q. My face is covered in freckles and I've always envied
people with pale skins, is there anything I can do?

A. You can make a milk bleach of an infusion of tansy mixed
with lemon juice. You'll find tansy growing in hedgerows
or in wasteground, with its big, feathered leaves standing
about two feet off the ground. It also has bright yellow,
flat-topped heads and there's an aura of camphor. But do
you really want to get rid of your freckles? They are so
pretty and youthful.

Q. Have you got any natural remedies for a hangover?

A. A Peruvian friend swears by this: take a whole cucumber
plus the skin, one apple and a cup of mineral water, put it
all in the blender and then drink it down. This is also a
good diuretic because it cleanses the system without
dehydrating you, unlike water pills.

Q. Models always look very slim, do you have to starve
yourself to stay this way?

A. Pat says: Not at all, I believe in eating a nutritionally-
balanced diet which contains plenty of vitamins and I
never feel hungry or skip meals if I can avoid it. Vitamins
are catalysts; for example an expert nutritionist told me
that if you combine orange juice and eggs, the Vitamin C
in the juice makes the iron in the egg yolks more readily
absorbed into the body.

Q. What is the best kind of comb to use so that my hair does not break?

A. A saw-cut comb is best; that means the edges of the teeth are flat and will not snag or pull your hair. Always use a very wide-toothed comb when combing through wet hair, so that you are less likely to break it—hair is in its weakest state when wet, so be gentle.

Q. Can you tell me how to make my own bath salts?

A. Pound in a bowl (a pestle and mortar are ideal but not essential) a packet of Epsom Salts with a few drops of food colouring and your favourite perfume or essential oil. Try yellow colouring with lemon oil, or green with pine. Do not put them in a stoppered bottle as they need the air to retain their colour—find a pretty dish and keep them near your bath. Not only are they decorative, but Epsom Salts help relieve muscular pain.

Q. When I put herbs in my bath water, they stick around the sides of the bath. Can I avoid this?

A. Place your herbs in the middle of a piece of gauze—gather up the corners and tie with a piece of string—or buy a metal tea-maker for one cup, and instead of putting in tea leaves, put in your herbs.

Q. What herbs can be used as natural colourants?

A. Camomile, marigold, rosemary, sage and rhubarb root are a few. Make infusions of the first four and a decoction of the rhubarb.
Camomile gives lights to blonde or brown hair.
Marigold gives a golden glow to fair hair.
Rhubarb Root is the strongest colourant and gives fair lights to blonde hair.
Rosemary lightens dark hair.
Sage darkens all hair and is particularly good for grey hair.

List of Shops

If you can't find any of the herbs yourself by browsing in the countryside, they can all be obtained from the following shops, to whom you should write with your requests:—

Baldwin & Co—173 Walworth Road, London SE17

Chalk Farm Nutrition Centre—42 Chalk Farm Road, London NW1 8AJ
(they also sell over the counter here)

Culpepper—Hadstock Road, Linton, Cambridge CB1 6NJ
(they have a retail shop in Bruton Street, London W1, and at Flask Walk, Hampstead NW3)

L'Herbier de Provence—341 Fulham Road, London SW10

Dr Malcolm Stuart—Albion Botanicals Ltd, 8 Grange Gardens, Cambridge

If you can't find what you want in your local chemist, a really good chemist where any of the oils and waxes can be purchased is John Bell and Croydon, 52 Wigmore Street, London W1H 0AU

Index